An Aztec Herbal
The Classic Codex of 1552

Translation and Commentary by
William Gates

Introduction by
Bruce Byland
Department of Anthropology
Lehman College and Graduate Center
The City University of New York

DOVER PUBLICATIONS
Garden City, New York

Bibliographical Note

This Dover edition, first published in 2000, is an unabridged republication of the work first published by The Maya Society, Baltimore, Maryland, in 1939. The illustrations reproduced in color in the 1939 edition are reprinted in black and white in the Dover edition. The Introduction was written by Bruce Byland for the Dover edition.

Library of Congress Cataloging-in-Publication Data

Cruz, Martín de la.
    [Libellus de medicinalibus Indorum herbis. English]
    An Aztec herbal : the classic codex of 1552 / translation and commentary by William Gates ; introduction by Bruce Byland.
       p. cm.
    Originally published: The De la Cruz–Badiano Aztec herbal of 1552. Baltimore : Maya Society, 1939, in series: Publication / Maya Society ; no. 23.
    Includes bibliographical references and index.
    ISBN-13: 978-0-486-41130-9
    ISBN-10: 0-486-41130-3
    1. Aztecs—Ethnobotany. 2. Materia medica—Early works to 1800. 3. Ethnobotany—Mexico. 4. Materia medica, Vegetable—Mexico. 5. Medicinal plants—Mexico. I. Gates, William, 1863–1940. II. Title.

F1219.76.E83 C78 2000
615'.321'08997452—dc21

                          00-024254

Manufactured in the United States by LSC Communications Book LLC
41130314   2021
www.doverpublications.com

Introduction to the Dover Edition

In May of 1990, Pope John Paul II made a pastoral visit to Mexico. In a conversation with the country's president, Carlos Salinas de Gortari, the Pope proposed that the Vatican make a momentous gift to the people of Mexico. He offered to return to Mexico the original manuscript of the *Libellus de Medicinalibus Indorum Herbis,* the first herbal and the first medical text known to have been written in the New World. This amazing and beautiful book had been written in Nahuatl, the Aztec language, at the College of Santa Cruz, in Tlatelolco, in the 25-year-old colony, called New Spain (now Mexico), by Martín de la Cruz, an Aztec physician. What Pope John Paul II was offering was not the Nahuatl manuscript, which is not now extant, but the Latin version prepared by de la Cruz's collaborator and translator, Juan Badiano, an Aztec nobleman and a professor at the College. It was that version that had been sent to Spain in 1552. There followed several years of incompletely documented meanderings before it became part of the library of Cardinal Francesco Barberini, the nephew of Pope Urban VII, early in the 17th century. In 1902 the Barberini library became part of the Vatican Library and there the "little book" sat until 1990.

Within the year, John Paul II presented the *Libellus* to the people of Mexico. After an absence of 438 years, this remarkable book came home. An invaluable piece of Mexico's intellectual and cultural patrimony had been returned to the land of its creation.

The *Libellus* has been known by several other names through the years. It is best known as the Badianus Manuscript, after its translator, or as the Codex Barberini, Latin 241, as it was catalogued by the Italian Cardinal who owned it in the 17th century. It also has been called the Codex de la Cruz–Badiano, after both its author and its translator. It is now most often known by its own original title, *Libellus de Medicinalibus Indorum Herbis.* It is in this way that this wonderful book is now catalogued in the library of the Mexican National Institute of Anthropology and History in Mexico City.

The *Libellus* was written in 1552 in Tlatelolco at the behest of the friar Jacobo de Grado, who was in charge of the Convent of Tlatelolco and the College of Santa Cruz. He, in turn, may have been working under the guidance of Fray Bernardino de Sahagún, the eminent Franciscan friar, and himself an author of many important studies of the Mexican people (cf. Sahagún

1950–69, 1986). De Grado had it written and translated into Latin for don Francisco de Mendoza, an advocate of the college and the son of the Viceroy of New Spain, don Antonio de Mendoza. Mendoza promptly sent it to Spain, presumably to the Hapsburg king, Carlos V, as evidence of the intellectual acumen of the Mexicans and in an appeal for support for the college. Germán Somolinos d'Ardois (1964:302–3) argues cogently that because of his troubles back home, Carlos V probably never saw the manuscript, but his son, who was later to be Felipe II, did receive it. Felipe relegated the manuscript to the royal library, where it was left virtually untouched. It contained much information about native curing practices, but it was not widely disseminated in Europe, perhaps because many of its ingredients were named only in Nahuatl, and were neither identifiable nor available in Europe. The manuscript was virtually unknown in Mexico, also, perhaps because it was sent to Spain so soon after it was written. It was not cited in any medical or botanical writing from either side of the Atlantic for the entire period from the 16th through the 19th century. That is not to say that its subject was not recognized. It was clearly appreciated as a beautiful and exotic work of art about medicine. We know that it came into the collection of Diego de Cortavila y Sanabria, the pharmacist to Felipe IV, king of Spain in the early 17th century. How it came to be in his possession is not known. From Cortavila it moved to Cardinal Francesco Barberini, perhaps directly or perhaps through one or more private collections, a transition that may have occurred when Barberini was in Spain during 1625 and 1626 (Vicario 1990:100). About this time, the only early copy now known was made by, or for, Cassiano dal Pozzo, who was an Italian bibliophile, a member of the Academy of Lincei, and a member of Barberini's mission. Rossella Vicario has found evidence of the creation of another Italian copy made at about this time by Francesco de' Stelluti, another member of the Academy of Lincei (Vicario 1990:100–1), but that copy is now lost. The dal Pozzo copy wound up in the collection of George III of England late in the 18th century and it, in turn, languished largely unnoticed in the library of Windsor Castle.

So things sat until 1929, when the *Libellus* was rediscovered. In that year Charles Upson Clark happened upon it in the Vatican library during a search for material related to the early civilizations of the Americas. In that same year Lynn Thorndike was reviewing the Barberini collection for documents related to the history of science and medicine. He noted the existence of the manuscript in his catalogue of Vatican manuscripts on the subject. Finally, also in 1929, Giuseppe Gabrieli published a brief note about the dal Pozzo copy that he had found some years before among the holdings of Windsor Castle.

William Gates seems to have learned of the manuscript from these first rediscoverers. He revived the moribund Maya Society in 1930 for the purpose of publishing his own writings when he became a research associate at Johns Hopkins University, and by 1931 the publication of the Aztec Herbal was planned. He received a complete set of photographs of the manuscript and watercolors of the botanical illustrations in 1932 and 1933 from Cardinal Eugène Tisserant, the Pro-Prefetto of the Library of the Vatican, and his niece, Marie Thérèse Vuillemin. He worked toward publication of the *Libellus* sporadically for the next seven years, completing various other projects in the meantime. Finally, in 1939, he published two volumes, one with the text in Latin and one with an English translation. What is here reproduced is Gates's 1939 English edition.

A simultaneous effort to produce an edition of the Herbal was being mounted by Emily Walcott Emmart, who also was associated with Johns Hopkins. Ms. Emmart learned of the manuscript in 1931 and, at the urging of many, set out to publish the Badianus Manuscript with a "facsimile, transcription, translation, and commentary" (Emmart 1940:ix). She, too, sought the aid of Cardinal Tisserant and his niece, who did the fine watercolors that Emmart ultimately published. A more accomplished scholar and a better fund-raiser, she was able, in 1940, to publish a skillful commentary and a full-color facsimile, together with many explanatory notes. Her English translation from the Latin is more fluid than is Gates's. Her edition was the only full-color facsimile published until 1964. Emmart's scholarship, though not beyond criticism, resulted in her work being widely regarded as "the most important English-language work on the Codex" (Foster 1992:14).

In the years following these early English-language editions of the herbal, one of the first things that a student will note is that the Badianus Manuscript has received all too little further study. Several facsimiles and a handful of analytical studies exist, but not nearly as many as would be expected to have come from the earliest complete medical text and the earliest herbal known from the New World. More commonly, the Badianus Manuscript is overlooked or is mentioned only in passing in a discussion of the colonial period in Mexico (cf. Gibson 1964:300).

The first published version in Spanish was presented in 1955 by Francisco Guerra in an extremely limited edition with very few plates (Guerra 1952). Parts of the commentary in this edition depended heavily on the work of Gates (Somolinos d'Ardois 1964:356–7).

The most important single later work on the manuscript is undoubtedly the Instituto Mexicano del Seguro Social edition of 1964 (de la Cruz 1964). This edition was the first widely available Spanish translation from the Latin and was published with a very good full-color facsimile, and several scholarly studies of various aspects of the manuscript and its contents. These include a very good study of the likely botanical identifications of many of the plants illustrated in the manuscript, by Faustino Miranda and Javier Valdés (1964:243–284). Similarly useful studies of the animals and of the rocks and minerals mentioned or illustrated are also included. An exceptional historical study of the manuscript was accomplished by Germán Somolinos D'Ardois (1964:327). Very good medical and dental studies are also included, as is a study of Nahuatl terminology done by Ángel Ma. Garibay K. (1964:359–374). A second edition of this work was issued in Mexico in 1991 in two volumes, one containing the text and another the facsimile (de la Cruz 1991).

A variety of specialized studies of the *Libellus* have been published since these major facsimiles and their accompanying analyses. What follows is a brief overview of some of these contributions.

Donald Robertson (1959:157) in *Mexican Manuscript Painting of the Early Colonial Period* noted that the manuscript represented a "meeting of two cultural streams—European science and native pictographic traditions." His concern was the identification and characterization of the Tlatelolco school of colonial manuscript painting as one of several colonial schools discernible today. The melding of European and native traditions in a seamless new form, so beautifully displayed in the Badianus herbal, is the hallmark of the Tlatelolco school. Robertson noted the use of native Mexican symbolic and iconographic representations presented in the context of the European herbal. He suggested that the author, Martín de la Cruz, the translator, Juan Badiano, and the unknown painter were heavily influenced by exposure at the college to European books and manuscripts. The mixing of the two traditions would have been an outgrowth of the general attitude of respect shown for native culture at the College of Santa Cruz, the first institution of higher learning in Mexico devoted to the teaching of native peoples.

X. A. Domínguez S. compiled a list of the plants identified in the manuscript by Gates (1939b), Emmart (1940), Reko (1947), and Miranda and Valdés (1964), and searched the chemical and pharmacological literature for studies of those plants (Domínguez 1969). For each of these plants he indicated the chemical constituents isolated from them and identified as pharmacologically active before the mid-1960s. This is an important contribution to ethnobotany, because Domínguez recognized the essential veracity of the medical prescriptions presented in the manuscript. The extent to which the prescriptions might work to cure or alleviate the conditions for which they are intended is not known, but the fact that they *could* work is suggested by the presence of pharmacologically active ingredients in the plants.

Debra Hassig (1989) published an excellent study of the three colonial Mexican herbals of the 16th century. The Badianus is the oldest of the three, followed by the herbal portion of Bernardino de Sahagún's Florentine Codex (1950–69: book 11, chapter 7) and the Historia Natural de Nueva España by Francisco Hernández (1959–84). She notes that, contrary to Emmart's view of its Mexican purity, the Badianus Manuscript displays pervasive indications of European medical practice, particularly of the medical "theory of humors" in which the four humors of the body (blood, phlegm, yellow bile, and black bile) must be maintained in balance. She also notes the Badianus' inclusion of the doctrine of "signatures," in which plants or other materials were judged appropriate to treat specific maladies because of clear physical similarities between the medicine and the condition. This, she asserts, was a borrowing from European medical traditions current in the 16th century. In this she is consistent with Robertson's view of mixed European science and native pictographic tradition. Hassig's analysis goes far beyond Robertson's simple view of the emulation of the style and form of European herbals by the authors of the Badianus manuscript. Hassig and Robertson essentially agree on this issue, but others have not shared the absolutist nature of their view, and would argue that much of what seems to them to be derived from European science could just as well be the product of native scientific traditions that parallel European ones in certain ways (see Furst 1995, Grivetti 1992).

Undoubtedly the most comprehensive and important study of Aztec medicine was accomplished by Bernard R. Ortiz de Montellano (Ortiz de

Montellano 1990). In a masterful study of the vast complexity of Aztec health and medicine, Ortiz de Montellano makes repeated careful reference to the *Libellus,* as, for example, in his initial discussion of the manuscript (1990:20–23). He points out that it was written for the purpose of demonstrating to the Spanish king the sophistication of his Aztec subjects and to show their familiarity with European culture. This observation leads Ortiz de Montellano to note that "the value of the Badianus as a primary source for knowledge of Aztec medicine is diminished precisely because of these efforts to show European sophistication" (1990:21). Separating Aztec medicine from European medicine, or from Aztec medicine distorted to emulate European medicine, is difficult under these circumstances. Nevertheless, he points out that for several ailments the treatments prescribed by de la Cruz are essentially the same as those prescribed in Sahagún, Hernández, or other colonial sources (Ortiz de Montellano 1990:159, 179). This is taken as an indication that for these diseases, at least, the *Libellus* is a reliable source for unadulterated Aztec medicine.

Louis Grivetti (1992) wrote about the Badianus manuscript as part of a wide-ranging study of the "prescientific origins of nutrition and dietetics." Grivetti focuses on the existence in the Badianus Manuscript of evidence of an allopathic medical theory that had much in common with the allopathy of many parts of the old world. Conceptually allopathy is embedded in the humoral theory central to 16th-century European medical practice. He also finds conceptual parallels with medical knowledge in China, India, and the Middle East. Central to allopathy in the Badianus manuscript, as Grivetti conceives it, is the well known "hot-cold" dichotomy in which bodily or spiritual imbalances in hot or cold are treated by rebalancing the body by application of the element lacking. Grivetti holds that this concept ". . . existed within the Aztec civilization . . . well before the arrival of the Spanish in 1519" (Grivetti 1992:16). This kind of parallel probably would be seen by both Robertson and Hassig as, at least partly, a product of European contact.

A brief discussion of the psychiatric ailments for which herbal treatments are offered in the Badianus manuscript and in Sahagún's Florentine Codex or *General History of the Things of New Spain* is provided by Guillermo Calderón Narváez (Calderón 1992, 1965). Calderón's discussion emphasizes psychiatric disorders that can be treated with plants that have a definable narcotic or analgesic effect. The idea that such disorders can be treated through drugs is, of course, an important part of modern medical practice.

Since the return of the Badianus manuscript to Mexico, two articles about it have been published, in 1992 and 1994, by Steven Foster in herb journals intended for a general audience. Accordingly, they are more advertisements for the 1991 edition of the book produced in Mexico than substantive treatments of its content. They include truly fine color reproductions of several pages of the manuscript.

Peter Furst recently published a remarkable study of the therapeutic qualities of psychoactive plants included in the *Libellus* (Furst 1995). He offers a thorough review and analysis of the identification and application in Aztec medicine of four psychoactive plants. These are various species of thorn apple *(Datura)*, the morning glory *(Turbina;* formerly *Rivea)*, cacao *(Theobroma)*, and tobacco *(Nicotiana)*. Following this discussion, he offers a well-thought-out consideration of the respective arguments of Hassig and Robertson concerning the degree to which the medical aspects of the herbal are derived from European sources. Furst concludes that the humoral theory that underlay so much of European medical practice of the time was readily adapted to Aztec medicine because it was inherently "compatible with the Aztec concept of the Universe ordered on a system of balancing opposites" (Furst 1995:126 citing Madsen 1955:138). Despite the apparent European references, the *Libellus Medicinalibus Indorum Herbis* appears to present a valid picture of Aztec medical practice complete with *materia medica,* formulae for use, and natural history of the pharmacopoeia. It is largely limited to these aspects of medicine, with relatively little inclusion of surgical treatment of injury and disease or of religious and magical aspects of medical treatment (see Ruiz de Alarcón 1982).

An illustration of the rising popular interest in this manuscript is the article about Aztec medicine published by Rob Nicholson in the December 1999–January 2000 issue of *Natural History* Magazine (Nicholson 2000). This small article, following in the tradition of Foster's essays, surveys several sources for the study of Aztec medicine but focuses on the Badianus as the earliest illustrated medical text from the new world.

The newer scholarly studies of the *Libellus Medicinalibus Indorum Herbis* can be seen as amplifications of the extraordinary work done by the first generation of students of this, the first medical text and first herbal of the new world. That newer studies have emerged is thanks, in large part, to the extraordinary scholarship of William Gates, Emily Walcott Emmart, and Francisco Guerra, in their early editions. It is my hope that this new publication of Gates's *Aztec Herbal* in an affordable and readily available form will inspire new studies of ethnobotany, new contributions to modern medicine based on the medical knowledge of traditional peoples, and a new appreciation of the great skill and inventiveness of Aztec medical practice in particular and Native American science in general.

Works Cited

Calderón Narváez, Guillermo

    1965   Conceptos psiquiátricos en la medicina Azteca contenidos en el Códice Badiano escrito en el siglo XVI. *Revista de la Facultad de Medicina.* México, D.F. 7(4):229–237.

    1992   La psiquiatría en el antigüo México. *Acta psiquiát. psicol. Am. lat.* México, D.F. 38(4):299–309.

de la Cruz, Martín

    1964   *Libellus de medicinalibus indorum herbis: Manuscrito Azteca de 1552: versión Española con estudios y comentarios por diversos autores.* Instituto Mexicano del Seguro Social, México, D.F.

    1991   *Libellus de medicinalibus indorum herbis: Manuscrito Azteca de 1552: versión Española con estudios y comentarios por diversos autores.* 2nd edition. Fondo de Cultura Económica and Instituto Mexicano del Seguro Social, México, D.F.

Domínguez S., X. A.

    1969   Algunos aspectos químicos y farmacológicos de sustancias aisladas de las plantas descritas en el Códice Badiano (Libellus de Medicinalibus Indorum Herbis). *Rev. Soc. quím. Méx.* 13(2):85–89.

Emmart, Emily Walcott

    1940   *The Badianus Manuscript (Codex Barberini Latin 241): An Aztec Herbal of 1552.* The Johns Hopkins Press, Baltimore.

Foster, Steven

    1992   The first herbal from the Americas: The Badianus Manuscript. *Herbal Gram* 27:12–17.

1994   The Badianus Manuscript: America's first herbal. *The Herb Companion* 7(1):27–33.

Furst, Peter T.
1995   "This Little Book of Herbs": Psychoactive plants as therapeutic agents in the Badianus Manuscript of 1552. In R. Schultes and S. von Reis, eds., *Ethnobotany: Evolution of a discipline.* Discorides Press, Portland, Oregon. 108–130.

Garibay K., Ángel María
1964   Nombres Nahuas en el Códice de la Cruz–Badiano. Sentido etimológico and Vocabulario de términos nahuas en el manuscrito. In *Libellus de Medicinalibus Indorum Herbis: Manuscrito Azteca de 1552: versión Española con estudios y comentarios por diversos autores.* By Martín de la Cruz. Instituto Mexicano del Seguro Social, México, D.F., 359–374.

Gates, William
1939a   *The de la Cruz–Badiano Aztec Herbal of 1552.* The Maya Society Publication No. 22, Baltimore.
1939b   *The de la Cruz–Badiano Aztec Herbal of 1552.* The Maya Society Publication No. 23, Baltimore.

Gibson, Charles
1964   *The Aztecs under Spanish rule: A history of the Indians of the Valley of Mexico 1519–1810.* Stanford University Press, Stanford, California.

Grivetti, Louis E.
1992   Nutrition past–nutrition today: Prescientific origins of nutrition and dietetics. *Nutrition Today* May/June 13–25.

Guerra, Francisco
1952   *Libellus de Medicinalibus Indorum Herbis: El manuscrito pictórico mexicano-latino de Martín de la Cruz y Juan Badiano de 1552.* Editorial Vargas Rea y El Diario Español, México, D.F.

Hassig, Debra
1989   Transplanted medicine: Colonial Mexican herbals of the sixteenth century. *RES: The journal of anthropology and aesthetics* 17/18 Spring/Autumn 30–53.

Hernández, Francisco
1959–84 *Historia natural de Nueva España.* 7 volumes. Universidad

Nacional Autónoma de México, México, D.F. Reprint of the work originally published in 1651 in a folio edition and later (1790) published in Madrid in a 3-volume edition with Latin versions of the botanical names.

Madsen, W.

1955   Hot and cold in the universe of San Francisco Tecospa. *Journal of American Folklore* 68:123–138.

Miranda, Faustino, and Javier Valdés

1964   Comentarios botánicos. In *Libellus de Medicinalibus Indorum Herbis: Manuscrito Azteca de 1552: versión Española con estudios y comentarios por diversos autores*. By Martín de la Cruz. Instituto Mexicano del Seguro Social, México, D.F., 243–284.

Nicholson, Rob

2000   Az-Tech medicine. *Natural History* 108 (10):54–59.

Ortiz de Montellano, Bernard

1990   *Aztec medicine, health, and nutrition*. Rutgers University Press, New Brunswick, New Jersey.

Reko, Blas P.

1947   Nombres botánicos del Manuscrito Badiano, *Sociedad Botánico de México* V:23–43.

Robertson, Donald

1959   *Mexican manuscript painting of the Early Colonial Period: The Metropolitan schools*. Yale University Press, New Haven, Connecticut.

Ruiz de Alarcón, Hernando

1982   *Aztec sorcerers in seventeenth-century Mexico: The treatise on superstitions by Hernando Ruiz de Alarcón*. Trans. and ed. by M. D. Coe and G. Whittaker. Institute for Mesoamerican Studies, Publication no. 7. State University of New York, Albany, New York.

Sahagún, Bernardino de

1950–69 *Florentine Codex: General history of the things of New Spain*. Ed. and trans. by C. E. Dibble and A. J. O. Anderson, 12 books. University of Utah Press, Salt Lake City, Utah.

1986   *Coloquios y doctrina cristiana*. Ed. and trans. by M. León Portilla, Universidad National Autónoma de México, México, D.F.

Schultes, Richard Evans, and Siri von Reis, editors

1995   *Ethnobotany: Evolution of a discipline.* Discorides Press, Portland, Oregon.

Somolinos d'Ardois, Germán

1964   Estudio histórico. In *Libellus de medicinalibus indorum herbis: Manuscrito Azteca de 1552: versión Española con estudios y comentarios por diversos autores.* By Martín de la Cruz. Instituto Mexicano del Seguro Social, México, D.F., 301–329.

Vicario, Rossella

1990   *Il Libellus de medicinalibus indorum herbis:* un erbario messicano del XVI secolo. *Arte Documento* 4:96–101.

PREFACE

The present volume contains the full text, in English version, with all the figures of the plants, as found in the original manuscript, which as Codex Barberini, Latin 241, has remained in the Library and archives of the Vatican since the time of that Cardinal Barberini from whom it holds its Vatican reference number, and of whose interest in the many forms of natural history much has come down to us, even including the naming after him of a magnificent cardinal-colored flower, by the botanists of his time. The manuscript itself was prepared as a tribute to the son of the then Viceroy of Mexico, in 1552, by two pupils, both then in the college at Tlatilulco; one of these, named Martín de la Cruz, having received his knowledge of medical plant values from the old men of his race, and to whom at base we owe the treatise; and the other, Juan Badiano, who owed his ' Latinity ' to the great Sahagún himself.

The manuscript is here published by The Maya Society through the good offices and authority of the present Cardinal Eugène Tisserant, at that time Pro-Prefect of the Library of the Vatican, on the occasion of his transmitting to us the complete set of photographs of the original, with a full set of most charmingly executed aquarelles of the plants therein shown, for our study and publication, made at the Pro-Prefect's instance for that purpose, by his niece, the Signorina Marie Thérèse Vuillemin, to both of whom our most grateful acknowledgments thus belong.

This was now nearly seven years ago, the actual publication having been put on our first list of agenda, following the incorporation of the Maya Society Foundation in 1931 for these purposes, and having remained on our own active list meanwhile. There have been delays, at times extended: the mere reproduction of the manuscript, however beautifully executed, and interesting, would have been little more than a collector's curiosity, in the almost total lack of attention among our scholars, north of the Rio Grande, or even knowledge of the existence of the great actual science of systematic botany and medical plant uses, in pre-Conquest days, long before Linnaeus' time. Thus the bare starting of the work, in a way worthy of the subject, and of ourselves as its sponsors, spread inevitably to bring in the section of Sahagún on medical and other plants, and the enormous work and records carried through and left for us by Francisco Hernández, still today almost unknown in this country; also therewith the clear data to be found in such pre-Conquest codices as the Mendoza and the Tellerio-Remensis. Then hunting through the bookshops abroad (useless a search in those of this country), for early works, rare in the extreme, and an extended literature in Spanish following, all took time, with delays and interruptions.

Elaborate indexes, of the Aztec terms and plants, of the Maya, of our own European botanical classifications, and of the classified diseases involved, had to be prepared. English translations, not only of the present little Herbal text, but of Sahagún and Hernández and other treatises, had all to be made, *and* made by the present writer in person.

These translations, indexes and appendant studies, all thus done some five and six years ago, have since lain while work on the parallel sciences of medical practice and plant knowledge among the Mayas, together with the coordination especially of the immense amount of like material gathered by the great Hernández from the same sources as those to which De la Cruz owed his skill and learning, went on under the Society's and my own personal aid and support at the Johns Hopkins University, following our receipt as above of these photographs and aquarelles. A very few Americans such as Mrs. Zelia Nuttall had in fact known of the actual existence of the manuscript, but it had not yet received the serious attention it does deserve for its contents and as a contribution to the History of Medicine, as well as for the beauty and skill of its colored plant pictures, then for the first time sent over to this country, for their inclusion, with the accompanying text, in our general series of works on pre-Conquest Middle America.

A complete but more compact edition of the text in Latin, with the drawings, was issued at the end of last year as our Maya Society Publication No. 22; in the present issue the original is followed page by page, in its order, but put into English, preceded by a brief survey of the science itself and further followed by an analytical index of the plants referred to, their nature and uses.

WILLIAM GATES.

The Johns Hopkins University,
    March, 1939.

Introduction to the Mexican Botanical System.

The plant kingdom was divided into two great natural Orders, the woody and the herbaceous. The term *quauh* ' wood,' applied not only to the tree as such, but to the hard woody part of any plant or bush, as well. The term *xiuh* ' herb,' applied to the lower plants themselves or to the soft herbaceous element; while the plural form *cuauhtla* denoted the ' woods ' among which plants were found growing.

The above trees and plants were then divided in four great artificial classes, according to their uses: edible, medicinal, ornamental and economic.

Each part of every plant being then subject to study and description, Families were formed based on the special characteristic quality of some type-member, just as with us. We thus have a *Xocotl, Tzapotl, Etl, Ayotl, Tomatl*-family; here the *xocotl* was taken as the ' type ' of acidulous fruits, the plum; the *zapote* of sweet fruits; then the Bean, Gourd and Tomato, our Leguminosae, Curcurbitaceae and Solanaceae, and so on.

Within these families were then ranged the different Genera, just as with us, the type-genus being one. Then as a natural consequence, not every Solanacea was a Solanum, any more than May-apples, pine-apples, custard-apples, love-apples, or *pommes de terre* are of a Genus ' Apple.'

It next became necessary to define the Species or individual, and if required its ' variations.' This was done by a true binomial nomenclature paralleling our own which began with Linnaeus, even to identity of terms in many cases. The type-form was further distinguished, naturally, by descriptive or determinative additions, constituting the second part of the binomial term. Of these two secondary parts, the descriptive terms form the natural classification, and the determinative the artificial; as we might say, ' bitter-root,' or else ' fever remedy,' ' Irish potato.' Exactly the same method is followed in our own Species glossology, save that while we do it popularly and regularly yet accurately, in the vernacular, our technical botanical terms we give in a Latin that carries their meaning far out of reach for the ordinary man. For the Aztec and Maya, this was not the case.

Also, as with us, while the nomenclature was effectively binomial, yet by compounding the second term it resulted in ternaries, and even in a few cases quinaries, owing to the extreme facility and richness of Aztec in word-formation and idea-incorporation. Thus while we say a Species is *erecta, repens,* etc. we also may say it is *albicaulis, trifoliata,* etc. And all these the Aztec names constantly reproduce in exact detail, in their Species definition.

For the development of this great system of classification and nomen-clature, every part of the plant, together with its various relations and likenesses, was studied and made use of. Apart from the four above major artificial Classes, the plant-world was described according to the way it was observed by our sight, taste, touch, smell, and even in the few such cases, as where it was *crepitans,* rustling, by our hearing.

This involved description by color, size, shape, surface appearance; as being sweet, acidulous, bitter, burning, salty; as feeling rough, smooth, rigid, hairy, furry; as smelling this or that.

The plant, whether tree or bush or herb, might be erect, drooping, prolate, creeping, climbing, winding, hanging, slender, spreading.

The habitat might be in cold regions or hot; in field, forest or garden; on stony soil, crags or walls; in marshes, water, by a riverside, seashore or by a still-water pond; here note the Aztec terms, *a-ten,* water-side, *a-toya,* running water, *a-tezca,* water-mirror or pool. Also geographical districts, by name.

The root would be straight, with edible tubers that are either like the camote or sweet-potato, or bulbous; or again bi-napiform.

The stalk would be knotty, resinous, etc.; the leaves round, dentate, ovate, palmate, digitate, spiculate. A conoid family would result with the Pine as type. Again a Grass family, a Cane family, and any of these natural characteristics used also to define species variations, exactly as with us.

The seasonal character of the plant, its times of maturity, would be one of the first things to be noted, and at times used in definition.

The economic values would result in such terms as paper-tree or plant; water-gourd, etc.

Finally the immense artificial Class of Medicinal plants would yield innumerable descriptive terms of primary value: pectoral, stomachic, diuretic, cathartic, emollient, stimulant, soporific, fatal, vulneraria, febrifuge, headache cure, cough cure, worm remedy, etc.; giving then the wholly invaluable pharmacological checks on correction of even the genera. It is from the nearly universal inattention to this angle that our mere formal taxonomic work limps so badly and produces such great confusion and many actual errors of classification, where various field gatherers have brought in multiple 'specimens' with different local names, usually misunderstood as to their meanings, or mistranslated.

It is to be noted that whereas Europe was brought out of its botanical depths by the *purely* artificial system of Linnaeus, which soon had to be modified and combined with natural classifications, in order to get any systematic nomenclature, the Aztec and Maya system—working from direct observation and on practical lines — from the first combined these two methods, the Artificial and the Natural, as above.

A combination of two distinct systems or methods necessarily results in duality of terminology, and in a Synonymy that is often exceedingly useful. The two terminologies must overlap; the natural characteristics give no indication of the artificial placements, nor the reverse. Whether a plant has tuberous roots or dentate leaves tells us nothing as to whether it is this or that disease remedy. Indeed, the same plant may be both alimenticious, curative and poisonous—as in the Solanaceae, and Marantaceae, and many others. The manioc gives poison for arrow tips, and sago for food.

Here then we have a system that is scientific and practical, and clear; definite and also expansible to any degree, as much as ours. For our study of this system we have divided the subject into its Classification, Glossology, Taxonomy, and Synonymy; but the Aztecs had still a fifth resource, which we lack.

Their science grew up and developed while they had painting and pictographic writing as their aids, only. All the names we have above referred to were those used in the spoken language, which was not written alphabetically. Their writing signs did not give the sounds of the words, but only the picture or idea of the thing.

This pictography was of two kinds, symbolic and natural or figurative. Now then the type-characteristic of the Family or other division was a condensed symbol, eliminating at times everything but the essential, as the conoid inflorescence of the pine, the red 'berries' of the tomato, etc. Color aided; tree-stalks would be brown, leaves green, desiccating grasses yellowish. The line between the artificial and natural, the symbolic and pictorial, followed over into this written memorial, to give a didactic-mnemonic science, using symbolic signs applied to plant groups, and various figurative determinants to denote the species. All this was then *matched* by the above synthetic incorporate words.

The town of Cuernavaca had to pay as annual tribute 160,000 sheets of paper, and other towns the like. Nothing is more historically certain than that we had here a great botanical descriptive literature. Sahagun tells us that none of his eight chief medical informants at Tlatilulco could "read," by which he certainly meant reading the alphabetic phonetic system introduced by the Spaniards. That they could take a compound pictograph such as the above, and give the corresponding term, the word, is certainly true. All of Hernández's information came from the skilled native informants, who knew their plants, their characters, synonymy, classifications, glossology and taxonomy—all of which he has given in his Thesaurus.

At his date these must have been chiefly men born before the Conquest; they must have derived their knowledge from the above pictographic-mnemonic-didactic system of transmission. Their predecessors had painted flowers on walls and sheets for the rulers and princes; had kept and developed these records for their own study.

One of these records we have in the priceless Codex Mendoza, with all its wealth of information on their life and customs. Among this we find typical plant drawings of which that of the pine, plate 41, fig. 8 may serve as illustration. This shows the tree in symbolic abbreviated form, as also constant elsewhere; the oblique striated lines, marking the appearance of the bark or (more probably) the cuts made on the trees for resin or turpentine; with a whitish appendix to the trunk that may denote the exuded resin itself; conoid elements, on the trunk and branches, and the parallel erect grass-like tip to the branches. This shows "a resin-producing tree, with conoid efflorescence and needle-like leaves," in short, a Pine. It was thus "readable" and translatable into our above botanic terminology. If further determinatives were needed, for any reason, they too could be added, and incorporated in the description, one part of which we put into our plant captions, and the rest extend in the text below.

As a necessary preliminary to a study of what the pre-Conquest Mexicans did in the building of their botanical science, we must understand and delimit strictly just what the Linnaean system is and does. It makes no attempt at a description of the plants themselves in their uses or general characteristics; it is something like a library shelf-finding system, referring any individual item to a particular wing, alcove or shelf.

It was added to, without being superseded, by the Jussieu and De Candolle 'methodic divisions,' based on the general characteristics. But even these latter only extend to the major Classes, and do not themselves go on to the descriptive terms of the innumerable genera and species, which at last do tell us what we really want to know about the plants, aside from their mere place-fixation in a system. The immense value of the Linnaean systematic classification, and the other methodic divisions, lies in their very neutrality, so to speak. They are neither Republicans nor Democrats, but only voters living at such a street and number.

Also, being general and neutral, they are comprehensive, and after the century and more of their use, have proven able to take in any and all newcomers, and give to each a definite and specific annotation, de visu the plant itself—that is, with its reproductive organs to go by. The three systems are therefore just as exact as the library reference number, or his formulae to a chemist. Of themselves they tell us nothing more. It was, in short, this very limitation of their scope that gave them their specific value.

What is of next importance to remember is that these systems did not in the least supersede the older methods of nomenclature, but only provided hooks to hang them on, as one comes to the Families, Genera and Species.

From time immemorial plants have been described and specified according to their appeal to our four senses, sight, taste, touch and smell; we still today find all these used in giving technical botanical names to species, and to a considerable degree to genera.

In addition to this, plants have been from the first described by terms telling their use, for the table or for the carpenter, or as curing this or that complaint. Our entire pharmacology follows this line: we speak of fever-remedies, diuretics, emollients, scab-cures.

A third element of definition is found in calling the plant after the place whence it comes: Michoacan root, jalapa, the China, Tabasco pepper; or again, more generally: mountain ash, rock-creeper, swamp-root, water lily.

A fourth appellative (naturally far less frequent in use) is in naming a plant after some particular person, whose memory is to be kept or honored; this is particularly true in the case of flowers, and in some cases of a remedy where the world owes that recognition to its discoverer.

Out of these four nomenclatures, as old as Eden and as modern as yesterday, has grown up a Synonymy which is at first a stumbling block to the novice, and later one of his most important doors to knowledge — as all stumbling blocks are. For we may find one plant called by any or all of the above terms, at once. Also, we may find several different botanical species (technically considered) using a like term. This does not necessarily imply an error by some one, but only that the person was not concerned with the technical taxonomic distinctions. Apples are apples, whether they are Snows or Winesaps, but neither pineapples nor May-apples are; the same also with the *tzapotl,* or *zapotes,* in old Mexico.

There are various plants that produce irritation of the skin on being touched; the giver of a taxonomic name may call any of them *urens,* so that we will get *Urtica urens,* etc., belonging to wholly distinct genera. In this manner a descriptive terminology is built up within and on the framework of the Linné, Jussieu and De Candolle systemic arrangement.

What is to be considered, as a preface to our coming studies, is that until the time of Linné an accurate and *informative* description of any plant had either to be given by a more or less compound term, or else to be reinforced by a sufficiently elaborate Synonymy. Given enough of these indications, the plant could be reliably defined. Linné made it possible to give every plant a systemic ' shelf-number.' All the old, necessary, descriptive terminology has still been kept, hidden by horrifying Greek and Latin extensibles — just as the Aztec physicians and herbalists did with synonymic equivalents they gave to Hernández. The only difference is that the Aztecs had not produced a Linnaean ' shelf-system.'

There is however a reason, perhaps, even for that. Men have always studied and had to study the plants by which they were nourished and cured; and we know absolutely nothing of how great was the antiquity from which this passage on of knowledge had come down, through Toltec and pre-Toltec times. But the Aztecs were tremendous lovers and students of plants and flowers of all kinds. They had great botanical gardens before Europe did; there was one a full league in extent on the Mexican plateau, and thereto came carefully wrapped tropical plants for study and care. Their empire itself was new on the highland of Anahuac, but it was spreading with all the concomitants of our European colonization of the past centuries. New plants and trade goods were as welcome in the Tianguiz or market place at Tenochtitlan as in London, Amsterdam or Sevilla. And with them came a Synonymy of place and kind and use that was, as Hernández's work clearly shows, a definite current factor in plant determination. His Indian instructors, as he fully confesses, gave him all this to make his great work possible; and without their contributions, and in a very large degree without this developed Synonymy, his monumental work would have been immensely less. They, the expert physicians and herbalists, were his direct dictating teachers, as they were of the priest Sahagún, and as we see shown in this small De la Cruz-Badiano manuscript Herbal.

On the other hand, although Hippocrates had himself stressed the value and necessity of Synonymy in the study of medical plants, Europe did nothing on that line until *after* Linné had produced his system. Lacking a working Synonymy, Europe was floundering, and needed Linné to pull it out and up. Mexico was utilizing Synonymy, as well as all the four descriptive methods we have above noted as being with us both pre- and post-Linnaean. All this then, so far as he could still gather it after the new Spanish era had come in and begun to overlay the old knowledge, driving it down into obscurity, Hernández got.

What now about Yucatan and the Mayas? First, in mainland Mexico we had the series of investigators and reporters of Spanish birth, chiefly Sahagún and Hernández; we had the school at Tlatilulco, where the little treatise herewith published was prepared, less as a scientific work than as an artistic and literary present to the Viceroy's son, but nevertheless an offshoot of the great, to us entirely new chapter in the History of Medicine and botanical discovery. We then for a time had continued activity in research under Spanish Mexican patronage and use.

For Yucatan we have neither Sahagún nor Hernández, but only Landa and Cogolludo, interested chiefly in religious matters and politics. The Maya were left to themselves, continued to *practise* the art of curing as it had come down for generations of their predecessors, father to son, *ah-tz'ac* to *ah-tz'ac,* and still preserved in our surviving corpus of medical texts, in the Maya language itself, and still awaiting its adequate translation and analysis. These texts in the Maya deal primarily with this direct medical practice, being captioned as such under the name of the ailment to be treated; while in Mexico proper, from Spanish pens, we have Latin treatises classifying and describing the plants themselves, as so captioned, in their botanical and incident pharmacological characters. Even the fountain-head there of all our knowledge, Hernández's work, with its 3000 names (reducible to some thousand actual plants) is no other than a mammoth Herbal, on Dioscoridean lines, mostly for Aztec and the plateau, but with Tarascan, Miztec or Huastec-named plants that had been brought in or reported to him.

Yucatan was thus a homogenous Maya unit, with its native skilled physicians and practical surgeons, now the long dead teachers of both ourselves and their present day inheritors and " keepers of the records." We are lacking here nearly all the aid of Synonymy given us for the expanding, commercial empire of Anahuac, with its constant incoming of new things from afar, and the consequent stimulation to interest and research, with the need for translating or explaining the foreign terms. But we still are left in the Maya with the other three of our nomenclature types, necessarily a part of the physician's practical knowledge, to assist our present understanding. Plants are given names descriptive of their appearance, taste, feel and smell; of their use for this or that, and as growing in this or that place, or position. In short, we have all the chief elements of *plant description*, whether that be Hippocratic, Apuleian, botanic and pharmacopoeic of today, Aztec, or Maya.

We have thus three coordinating factors to carry us forward in our present work: physical plant description, medical use, and the science of linguistics. These three interlock, and cross-check. For the Aztec side of the matter, very extensive and able work has been done by Mexican scholars, and ignored by us (for that reason); our English writers are hardly even acquainted with the very name of Francisco Hernández, who was nevertheless one of the greatest exploring and research scientists, in the truest sense of that word, that ever left European shores. Absorbed in the sudden expansion of our bacterial and serum advances, and synthetic remedies, we have forgotten that through the sheer hard force of necessity, plus the exploring urge that is man's very nature, people have studied and been cured through the ages.

Also, none of us know either Aztec or Maya, and most of us think of those as dead languages, and their knowledge as superstition. To this we add the utterly illogical and groundless theorem that " medicine has grown out of and is deeply rooted in superstition and magic," magic being a convenient term for still un-rediscovered science.

The present pretends to be no more than an " *Introduction* to the pre-Conquest Aztec Botanical System "; and as such we must needs give the reader enough extended instances of its synonymy, glossology, iconography and taxonomy to outline its methods and scope. What ought to be done should be to give to scholars a full edition in English of the hundreds of closely printed folio pages of the Hernández " Thesaurus," with all its illustrations; a mere listing, as here follows, of classified botanical terms, with their meanings and uses, must suffice us, fairly to cover the above headings. Yet even so, the detail and scope of the system, the careful observation and the accuracy of the descriptions on which the whole was based and developed, are manifest, and shown in no small degree in this work of Martin de la Cruz, practical plant knower and artist, and his translator Juan Badiano, the Latinist.

The names or items have been taken, as they came, from either the original folio edition of 1651, or from the much expanded text first published in 1790, long after the author, back in Spain, had recast his original Dioscoridean order into practical agreement with the " natural " Mexican system. The reader must then, at the start, remember that each of the following items is, in the original Latin text of Hernández, accompanied by long descriptions, often over a page in length, of the plant itself, its habitat, uses and synonyms.

Synonymy.

Toto-ycxitl, bird-foot, has the limbo deeply split, in five principal lobules; it was further called Caxtlatlapan, placing it in the Convolvulaceas, to which it clearly belongs, being an Ipomoea. Two names, vulgar and scientific.

Chucté, Huastec, Huitziloxitl in Aztec, of the Leguminosa.

Tzitziqui, Tarascan, *Huitzo-cuilcuitlapil-patli* in Aztec, of the Composites.

Chapol-xochitl, locust-flower; also *Tenapalitl*, or siempreviva, an indication for phytography, and also for its classification; further called *Minca-patli*, arrow medicine, to cure wounds; also *Comal-patli*, spleen medicine, and so used. In Tarascan, *Pinipiniche*.

Itzmi-quilitl, vegetable or edible plant like an obsidian knife, *itzmitl*, from the form of the leaves, but also indicating a portulaca. Also *izta-quilitl*, salty vegetable, and *tlal-izta-quilitl*, creeping salt vegetable. *Quilitl* is an artificial classification for all garden plants; *tlal*, from *tlalli*, denotes any low or creeping plant, a *rastrera*.

Oco-petlatl tepiton, which is the same as Helecho small; also *huapaz-patli*, compact medicine, for cramps; finally *i-tzinpech-tetl, basim lapideam*, plant with stony base, i. e. growing on stony ground. (See several such shown iconographically in the Badiano.)

Of all our given 3000 names, 250 are Tarascan, with which region our author had direct contact; 36 plants from the Mizteca have only their Aztec rendered name; only 3 are Miztec; a very few are Huastec; none have brought Zapotec, Totonac or Matlalzinca.

Poztec-patli, fracture remedy; in Otomí, *Tunqui-yeti*, from *ton*, break, *yethi*, medical plant.

Mexican nouns regularly have the ending *-tl* added to the root or stem. *Quahuitl* is tree or wood, *quauh-* as prefix is the radical, also used to denote a plant growing wild, ' in the woods,' the same as the Maya *che*, tree, or also *kax*, forest, *monte*. *Xihuitl*, stem *xiuh*, means an herbaceous plant, also the non-woody part of a large tree or bush, the branches; Molina defines it as *ramos de árboles*, the ' plant of a tree.' We now have:

Mica-quahuitl, death-tree, an arboreal Convolvulacea; *mica-xihuitl* seems to be a Lobelia.

Quaquauhtzin means any bush, arbuscula; *qua* being the radical of *quaitl*, the top or head, *-tzin*, a word-ending meaning small; thus ' small tree top.' Then *ahuatzitzin*, small oak; *tepe-chichian-tzin*, small wild, or mountain, *chian*; *copal-tzin*, small copal; *meme-tzin*, small maguey, *quauh-xiuh-tlepatli*, burning frutescent medicine, using *tletl*, fire, *patli*, medicine.

In describing the form the ending *-tic*, ' like,' is mainly used as we use the Greek eidos; *chichiantic*, to compare the plant with a Verbenacea, *herba similis chian*. Also used in the same sense *-to*, *-ton*, *-tzin* to give the idea of likeness or affinity. In popular speech *-yo* is also common, forming an adjective: *atemitl*, *atemyo*, lousy, *iztlacti*, *itzlactiyo*, poisonous. Thus we have the names *chian-tzotzol-to*; *popozo-ton*; *ato-tzin*; *ahuahuauh-yo*, plant like the Bledos.

When we come to denote the nature of the ground or soil; *atl*, root *a*, is used as prefix to aquatic plants: *tentli* bank, *a-ten*, by the side of water; *tezcatl*, mirror, *a-tezca*, beside still waters; *a-toyatl*, by a river or running waters; *atl-i-nan*, mother of water (perhaps as shading it; *a-pan-choloa*, what leaps from water, a Cuphea, belonging to very moist places; *atlan-chane*, dweller of the waters, another Cuphea; *a-ten-xihuitl*, plant on banks of rivers, compared with the Laver or Sium, of the Umbelliferas; *tlal-atez-quilitl*, a short stemmed pool grower, said to be like the Berro, Cruciferas; *atoya-xocotl*, acid river plant, a Spondia, Terebinth; *a-xochi-atl*, using the water root twice, for our Senecio vernus, a Spring plant, beginning to flower with early rains, and stopping when they are full.

For stony ground we have *tetl,* stone, root *te;* then *tetla* for stony place; *texcalli, texcal-,* crag; *tepetl, tepe-,* mountain, in the same way that the Spanish *monte* has come to be the specific word for woods or a wilderness; *tetl-i-pepech,* blanket of stones; then *te-nochtli,* stone cactus, as seen in the Mexican coat of arms, and also the old name of the city, Tenochtitlan; *texcal-amatl,* a fig growing on crags; *tepe-cimatl,* mountain root, a Leguminosa growing in mountains in the hot lands, as the *quauh-cimatl* is another Leguminosa growing in woods on the borders of the hot lands; again the *quauhtla-huitzitzil-xochitl,* wood-flower of the humming-bird, growing in shady forest places.

The word for sand, *xalli, xal-* also gives us the *xal-temecatl,* or *xal-quahuitl,* growing by running water.

As names for the different parts of the plant we have *nelhuayotl,* the root, the foundation or beginning of something; *quahuitl,* the woody stem; *quauh-xihuitl,* the herbaceous part, the branches; *quauh-atlapalli,* the leaves; *xochitl,* the flower; *xuchi-qualli,* the fruit, or ' good to eat ' part. The particular form of the root may be known by the term *cimatl,* for roots nearly always crass, perpendicular, and at times pivoting; if a tuber it is a *camotli,* or if round, orbicular, *xicama, xicamitl,* as the dahlia, a Composite. From this we get *cima-patli;* also *cicimatic,* a bi-napiform root; the *xicamatic,* non-edible.

Edible *camotes* are the sweet potatoes, Convolvulacea; *cacamotic-tlanoquiloni* was a purgative, tuberous, *camote; quauh-camotli,* or yucca, a manihot, with fecula and edible, *Euphorbiacea.* The modern term *camote de cerro* may be the *tepe-camotli,* of the Dioscoraceas. When, after the Conquest, the white potato, Solanum tuberosum, came in, the natives called it *pelon camotli,* or Peru potato.

Among the Trimetra, Composites, with their rhizome tubercles, we find the *atepo-patli,* or ' tadpole ' remedy. Probably among the Polygonaceas we have the *ilahcatziuhqui,* or twisted thing.

Classification.

The Indian Classification was of two sorts, interwoven: Natural and Artificial. Their division first into the great natural Orders of Trees and Herbs was fundamental; these names referred not only to appearance, but to their consistence and duration; *xihuitl* is also the word for year, and hence perhaps implied the idea of the ' annuals '; it specifically meant not only the low or herbaceous plants as such, but the herbaceous parts of a tree, until these passed into woodiness, the hard state.

Next after these major Orders, we have an artificial division into the four Classes, the food plants, the medicinal, the flowers and the economic. The first three of these being both distinct and numerous, they have the general Class-names, *quilitl, patli, yochitl*, always the final member in their descriptive terms. The economic Class lacks a similar single Class-term to distinguish their broad use as such. The four classes, standing thus between the Orders and the next subordinate division, the Genera as such, function in a way as Genera, but lack the botanical, or taxonomic meaning and value.

The fourth level of subdivision is that of the Genera, and then the fifth, the Species, strictly comparable to our own classificatory use of these terms. Thus we have many genera, marked or named by their type-form, as with us the pod type including both the pea vine and the locust tree, the Tomato genus or Solanacea, etc. One such wide Genus among the Aztec has as its type the 'cord' element, *mecatl*, and including generically Enredaderas, Trepadoras, Bejucos or vines, Sarmientos.

Among these *mecatls* we thus find: the Smilax; the *cozol-mecatl* or cradle vine; *meca-patli,* medicinal vine, and the *quauh-meca-patli,* a wild variety; the *meca-xochitl* (see the Badiano, p. 104), with the marks of a Piperacea; *coa-mecatl,* snake cord, of the Polygonaceas; the *te-mecatl* is an Ipomoea, of the Convolvulacea; another *meca-patli* is a voluble, of the same family; the *colo-mecatl, colo-te-mecatl, colo-mecatl-xihuitl,* an Ipomoea; another *te-mecatl,* from Yauhtepec, a climber with tendrils, perhaps a Bryonia; *qua-mecatl latifolia* and *tenuifolia,* the seeds compared with Phaseolus, are Leguminosae; the same perhaps of the *iztac-mecatl,* or ' white cord '; *xoxo-mecatl,* our Parra silvestre; a third *te-mecatl* may be a Cissus, Ampelidacea; *quauh-mecatl,* Serjania mexi-cana, a woody plant, probably trepadora of the Sapindacea; and finally the *te-qua-mecatl,* placed by the Linnaeans in the Clematiceas.

Among the *patlis* is the *itzquin-patli,* dog-bane, exactly our Senecio canicida, of the Composites; also *quimich-patli,* rat poison. In all these *patlis* we find just as with us, so that they may be named, e. g. as giving heat when that is needed, or reducing it for a fever; a '-moisture'-*patli* may check or increase that, as called for.

The alimentation, especially of the lower classes, was chiefly in herba-ceous plants, wild or cultivated. These again formed a large artificial group, the *quilitl,* the garden or edible plant. Their enumeration would be interminable, and so just a few here.

The *tlan-epa-quilitl,* fox-tooth vegetable, Piperacea; *chichic-quilitl,* the *yerbamora,* a Solanum; *huitz-quilitl,* and a wild variety, *qua-huitz-quilitl,* usually looked on as being thistles (see the Badiano, p. 73), but being certainly edible, should be referred to the Alcachofas, Cynara, Cinareas; *acoco-quilitl,* with a fistulous stem, of the Umbelliferas; *itzmi-quilitl,* with various synonyms, our verdolaga, Portulacas; *cochiz-quilitl,* a soporific for children, an Erythrina.

The ornamental plants, the flowers or *xochitl,* made another grand division, often with definition of the odor, although beauty was the desired feature, even with no odor. Among these are *xochi-quahuitl,* Cordia odoratissima, whose wood smells like cologne; *tona-xochitl,* heat flower, the spadix heating during fecundation; *huacal-xochitl* (see Badi-ano, p. 30), an offering to the gods and the monarch, compared to a Dranunculus; the *atzcal-xochitl,* rose-colored, compared with the sea-oyster; the *ocelo-xochitl,* or tiger flower, Tigridia.

Among the orchids, *coa-tzonteco-xochitl,* snake-head flower, an An-guloa; another is yellow, the *coztic-coa-tzonteco-xochitl,* of the Sobralia.

Among the aromatics, the Labiadas, we find the *olo-xochitl,* with spiciform inflorescence; also the *cuitla-xochitl,* perhaps a Verbenacea. Also the Myrtaceas, aromatic, the *xoco-xochitl,* acid flower, a Eugenia.

The *totec-y-xochiuh,* assigned to the Heliotropium, and meaning the flower of Totec, or God our Lord. The Plumeria was greatly esteemed, the rubra being the *cacalo-xochitl,* crow flower, and alba the *tiza-xochitl;* the *tlapaltic-cacalo-xochitl* was reserved for the monarchs and grandees.

Among the Rubiaceas, the *tlaco-xochitl,* a Bouvardia, was brought from the west coast to Anenecuilco in Morelos, for its tonic and medicinal qualities.

Of the Cacti: the white *nopal-xochitl;* the finest of all the yellow *coztic-xochitl.* (We have also a medicinal *coztic-tomatl,* yellow tomato.)

The *chamol-xochitl* is the Poinciana pulcherrima; the *mapil-xochitl,* finger flower, of the Bombaceas; and finally the *cacahua-xochitl,* or cacao flower, Lexarza funebris.

Taxonomy.

In the Indian nomenclature the adjective or qualifier precedes the substantive, as we say cultivated hemp and not *cannabis sativa,* creeping tulip, not *tulipa repens.* The last member of a compound Aztec term represents the genus, and is connotative, giving the dominant charac-teristic, and thus the basis of the Classification. It thus also retains the final *-tl* of the Aztec noun, while all the preceding species qualifiers, limiting as adjectives the final element of the term, lose the *-tl* and show only the simple stem, as *quauh* instead of *quauhtli; acatl* is a cane, but *aca-zacatl* is cane-grass. As seen in the pictorial nomenclature, we find the major groups shown by this final member as giving us the Orders, Genera and Species, each developing the lower members of the class by these adjectival descriptives, exactly as we do, save that the Aztec word order of the compounds is as in English, not the Latin. Thus we get such a completely indicative term as *Tepe-huil-aca-pitz-xochitl,* ' mountain-flute-cane-tall-flower,' a voluble Bignonacea, or jas-mine; as *huilaca* is the word for flute-cane; and *pitzli* means tall.

Huaxin, pod, *Mizquitl,* legume, *Etl,* seed of a legume, *Huacalli,* stri-ated thing, *Coyolli,* rattle, *Tecomatl,* vase, are thus Genera, while the species name referred to the kind of soil or habitat, to some attribute of the plant, its form, consistence, coloration, direction, or other;

not infrequently its use was noted, or the name of some similar or related plant employed.

We may as illustration take one generic group, with its species, that of the rushes, *espadaña*, our Tule, in Aztec, *Tollin*. There were many others, not only in this group, but in the immense group of the Mono-cotyledones. Note Sahagún's *a-itz-tollin*, using *itzli*, flint, for sharp leaves that cut when grasped; *tepe-tollin*, mountain reeds; *tlil-tollin*, black reed; *tzon-tollin*, hairy reed; *ix-tollin*, for ophthamia, from *ixtli*, eye; *cal-tollin*, for use in the house; *calli*; *petla-tollin*, for making mats; *a-tollin*, aquatic; *nacace-tollin*, triangular; *popo-tollin*, broom-tule, Sco-parius; in all these the *tollin* being the genus.

In the adjectival position we again have: *tol-cimatl*, tule root, *tol-patli*, tule remedy. But in these the *cimatli*, *patli* mark a higher Class-grade, *cimatli* being applied to any plant with large roots, and *tolcimatl* of the Ciperacea being thus matched with *ayeco-cimatl* of the Le-guminosa.

Patli now is the general term for all remedies or medicinal plants, so that there must be many *patli*: *tol-patli*, *quequexquic-patli*, *chian-patli*, of the Ciperaceas, Araceas and Labiadas. In a like way we have *tol-patlactli*, ' broad tule thing,' *tol-mimilli*, column of tule. Thus we may consider *patli*, *cinatl*, *patlactli*, *mimilli* as *officinalis*, *macrorrhizus*, *latfolium*, *teres*, *rotundus*, *cylindraceus*, etc.

The above terms are binaries, *a-itz-tollin* a ternary, just as we have Beta vulgaris rapacea. Then *iztac-xoco-nochtli*, white cactus fruit. Again a variety, or even a distinct species is marked by a separate added word, as *atoya-xocotl chichiltic*, red river-fruit; *te-copal-quahuitl pitzahuac*, or a copal-tree tenuifolium.

The one great defect in any system not involving the purely formal, non-descriptive Linnaean, is the inevitable repetition of names, as we have our innumerable ' cough medicines,' ' female remedies,' etc. This is particularly the case where the term is therapeutic. Thus there are 37 *iztac-patli*, white medicines, and 21 *cihua-patli*, the name given to all uterine, etc., remedies. Of the *palanca-patli* (the *ķaaķ-tz'acob* in the Maya), there are 13. And in such cases Hernández constantly added terms of his own, either descriptive, place, or those of the earlier European botanists; but these were not altogether with -patli terms. Thus he calls six different plants chichiantic, ' like the chia,' all six here being from different places; what was probable here is that a local plant found to have the qualities of that in the central Anahuac region, got its name applied, as in the case of the Salvia chian. A multiplicity of synonyms is necessarily an incident of the place or time equations, as where the Ximénez Spanish version of Hernández, done forty years later, twice has synonyms added, not in the Latin version. Lacking the specific Linné identifications, synonymy is the taxonomic make-weight; thus we find tecomahaca also called copal-ihyac, smelling like copal, which helps much since copal is used for many Terebinths.

Thus also the nacaz-colotl, twisted ear, now called cascalote, was recognized by Humb-B. as Caesalpina cacaloco, Leguminosa, and then by them given the regional name.

It is just here that our modern Taxonomic science limps so badly, from our failure to include all three essential factors to identication; the physical ' specimen ' in a folder, pharmacological attention and, in foreign sources, the almost universal ignorance of the local language, to check and understand the innumerable blind synonyms worked out by the gatherer in situ.

Glossology.

To give the reader a fair idea of the accuracy and spread of the system, from the purely botanical standpoint, some statement in detail of the terms employed and their constantly close correspondence with our own, is essential. The present is only meant to be an Introduction to the science, and mere space reasons forbid more than a running selection of the terms we find in use. Quite a few of these will be found in the iconographic pages following, even, fortunately, including a number of the various plants pictographically represented by De la Cruz in our short herbal. A great help will be also in the extended list of place names glyphically shown in the Mendoza and Tellerio-Remensis pre-Conquest codices. The 1651 folio Hernández, with its hundreds of illustrations, is effectively a great Herbal; but our most direct aids will be found in the 3-volume Madrid edition of 1790, with its Latin-rendered Aztec names. Our references below will be to volume and page of this edition, starting as above noted with the primary size and substance of the plant world: the tree, *quahuitl;* herbaceous plant, *xihuitl;* bush, *quaquauhtzin.* From there we shall take in order the different plant parts and elements of description, taking over the old order Latin terms used by Hernández without attempting their present-day revision, which we most willingly leave to the taxonomic specialists.

Quaquahtzin is a bush, arbuscula, *qua* being the radical of *quaitl* the top or head and *-tzin* the diminutive ending; thus a small tree with spreading top. Again we have *ahua-tzitzin,* small oak; *tepe-chichian-tzin,* small mountain or wild *chian; copal-tzin,* small copal; *copal-quahuitl,* i-359 is a tree Terebinth, *copal-xihuitl,* i-365 an herbaceous Labiada. Here we may also note the *qua-quauh-xochitl,* bush flower, a Cereus.

Quahuitl may also denote dryness, for which see the Molina diction-ary; then the maize stalk *ohuatl,* when it goes dry becomes *ohua-qua-huitl;* the tall stalk of the maguey, *quiotl* or *xiuh-quiotl,* when dry be-comes *quio-quahuitl.* As the green herbaceous parts become dry, woody and hard, they are then *quahuitl.* Next, from the root *ma* we get both the words *maitl,* arm or hand, and *matia,* to branch out; thus the first subdivisions from the stem, at times mere leaves coming out direct, are the *xiuh-maitl,* and *i-mama-in-quahuitl* the arms of the tree; then while *mo-xiuh-yo-tia* is to put out the herbaceous green leaves, *qua-quam-ma-tia* is to put out branches high up, or at the top. Also finally bringing in the scabby eruption *xiotl,* as a descriptive terminal we have *copal-quauh-xiotl,* i-367, a Terebinth, a Rhus.

Here we can note the bark, or skin, *ehuatl;* and if this skin grew in character as such, we get *cempoal-ehuatl,* 20-skins, or elm. From this going on to other qualities of the stem: the surface, length, coloration, composition, form, etc.

The *pepeyo-quahuitl,* as the álamo, shining.

The *tohmiyo-xihuitl,* ii-367, plant covered with soft down; see our Herbal, p. 111.

From *tzontli,* hairs, *quauh-tzontli,* i-82.

From *tezontli,* a rough stone, *quauh-tezon-quilitl,* iii-122, a rough-barked edible. A rough skin may also be called *xal-quahuitl,* sandy, iii-339, at the same time as the *xal-tomatl* is a plant with tomato-like fruit, growing in sandy soil.

From *huitz,* spine or thorn, we get many names: *huitz-quilitl,* the cardo or edible thistle; *huitz-tomatzin,* ii-6, small spiny tomato, or Sola-num Hernandezii; the Acacia albicans with its many thorns and geminate, i-262, the *huitz-ixachin-quahitl.* If the thorns are very hard, prefix the *te-* of *tetl,* for an acacia of the Leguminosaš, *te-huitztli.*

Tlal, from *tlalli,* earth, not only means a low ground plant, or any ' low ' plant or variety (as our pea-vine is a ' low ' pod plant, against the tall locust with its pods), but may also mean just short-stemmed, as the *tlal-omi-xochitl,* a lily, iii-45.

If the plant is tall, ' long,' add the adjectival *piaztic, piaz-tlacotl,* said to be slender and five cubits high: 1651 ed., p. 399.

If simply slender, the *te-xiu-pitzahuac,* with stringy roots, caulibus strigosis, ii-472.

If cylindrical, or round like moon or shield, *tlaco-yayahual,* ii-463, virga rotunda.

From *nanace,* an angle, the *nanacace,* iii-22, assigned to the Cynareas, if 4-sided, use *nahui-teputz,* with four shoulders; again *nahui-y-nacaz,* 4-cornered.

To describe the globular stem of the cactus take the word *comitl,* a vase: *tepe-nex-comitl,* a mountain plant with ashy colored potato-like root, defined by Candolle as an Echinocactus.

A geniculated stem, the *tlatlanquaye,* or plant with knees; see the 1651, p. 210, an Amaranth.

If the stalk bends like the handle of a jar, or with bending branches like the weepers, use *hui-collotl.* If voluble, enwrapping, use *mecatl,* rope; see the *meca-xochitl,* cord flower, the Piper amalago, a flowering plant with voluble stem. For our rastrera or humifusa, *tlalli* (ground-clinging), or *huila,* lame and creeping, as *huilanqui,* ii-351.

According to Molina *tetepuntli* is a truncated stalk and *ma-tetepun* a hand cut off; then *tetepuntic-quahuitl,* trunk of cut down tree, and *quauh-tetepuntli,* a stick fastened in the ground; *coa-cuitla-tetepon,* spinal column of snake, the axis like the Triticus repens. *Maxac* is a crotch, *maxacaloa,* to put out branches, leaving the *tete-puntli* the simple stalk without branches or leaves.

Taking now the leaves: *maitl* is the hand or branch, and *quil-maitl*, the ' green arm ' of an herb, giving us a veritable axillary system, primary, secondary and tertiary, from the *tetepuntli* to the leaves. These latter are more specifically the *atlapalli*, the thoracic branches, the ' wings,' *xiuh-atlapalli* or *quauh-atlapalli*.

Then for the composition, they counted the number of leaflets that received the nervations of the common bud; for the compound leaves of Phaseolus, pinnate, *etl* or the number three was used as we do trifoliate. In some places they are still today said to call a Tecoma, Bignoniaceae, a quinque-foliate, *macuile*, from *macuilli*, 5; also *macuil-y-ma*, iii-416, the 5 of the hand, from the disposition of the leaves.

For verticillate leaves use the term ' bird's foot,' *totol-icxitl;* see 1-63, *acatzana-icxitl*, thrush-foot. If we complete the name *toon-chichi*, ii-9, a geminate Solanum, by adding *tomatl*, the generic for many Solanaceas, then (*toon*, *to-ome*, equalling 2 x 2), we have a bitter tomato with geminate leaves.

For sessile, knotty, fistulous, use the *acatl*, or cane: 1651 ed. pp. 262, 263, *aca-coyotli* and the *aca-xaxan*, with knots and alternate subsessile leaves.

For the peduncle other terms, with qualifiers for the leaf. Then for the limbo the term *ixtli*, face: *ix-matzal*, ii-372, deeply divided; *ix-patlahuac*, ii-374, broad; *ix-pipitzahuac*, ii-378, narrow; *ix-nexiuhqui*, ii-466, ashy stalk and under surface; *ix-cuicuil*, ii-371, painted, compared by Hern. with the Rutacea, many of which have translucent spots; *ix-tenextic*, ii-373, limelike whitish; *ix-tezontic*, ii-374, rough; *ix-tomio*, ii-367, hairy or furry; *ix-yayahual*, limbo orbicular, as compare the Cochlearia crucifera, see ii-461, 462; also compared with the fronds of Adiantum; *tepan-ix-yayahual*, ii-463, or literally ' parietaria de limbo orbiculare,' *tepan* meaning wall.

For the leaf nervation, terms rendering digitinerve, palmatinerve, peltinerve, using *macpal* for palm of the hand; *macpal-xochitl*, or Cheirostemon, palmati-lobate. Then when the fig was introduced it was at once called *macpal-quahuitl*, for its palmatinerve limbo. Finally, for the term *peltinerve*, *tzinacan-atlapalli*, iii-453, the bat-wing.

In all such names we will note not geometrical terms, or such as ' circular,' but some known observed object, as a table; for pointed ovoid,

like a rabbit's ear; if very narrow, like hairs, and if very short like eye-
lashes; *huey-tochtli-nacaztli*, ' big rabbit's ear,' seems to be an Asclepias
cornuti; *tzon-metl*, i-81, compared with Daucus of the Umbelliferae, for
the pinnati-secta and almost lineal divisions; and *ixquamol*, a bush ii-371,
eyelash plant. If cordiform, note the *yollo-chichiltic*, red-heart, i-42,
giving both form and color.

For serrate there are various terms, at times comparing with the oak;
again use *tzitziquil*, split, or *tlan-tectli*, tooth-cut; *chichic-ahauzton*, 1651
ed. p. 143, Dipsacus, bitter plant with serrate leaves. If the limbo is
more deeply split, compare with an animal's hoof for our terms multifid,
trifid.

For the color, only abnormal colors are noted, as *tlil-quahuitl*, iii-218,
blackish purple; *nenexton*, at iii-6 compared with Siempreviva, Crasu-
lacea; also see our Herbal for *nexehuac*, ashy plant, and almost certainly
being Datura inermis. At page i-34 we find described a plant with two-
colored petals, blue and red, and the leaves green on one side, blue the
other. *Xaxahuactli*, iii-350, is a ' painted plant,' while the *tetl-y-xahual*,
iii-249, is a painted plant growing on stones, its leaves tending to gold.

If the leaves are thick and fleshy, they are *nahui-y-tilma*, ' four-
mantled,' iii-11. The *nahui-tlaquen*, ii-475, is said to have four tegu-
ments, and related to the Aizoon, of the Ficoideas. If the limbo is rigid,
use again the *te* of *tetl*, *te-atlapalli*, stone-wing, i-217, assigned to Adiantum. *Zaca-papalo-quilit*, edible pasture with very delicate leaves, *papalo*,
a butterfly.

Iconography.

The key to the system and the effective study of Botany, whether
European or Mexican, lies in the divisions of the plant world into
families and genera, defined by some major characteristic shown in common. These divisions and characteristics are then set forth by the
definitive or descriptive terms used, as covered in the preceding section,
the Glossology, whether Latin or English, or Aztec.

The Mexicans, however, did not set down on paper their spoken
words, names, verbs or other parts of connected speech, in alphabetic

characters standing for the spoken sounds, but in symbols representing the things or ideas involved. Their writing (and they had it in full sense) was Ideographic or when relating to physical things seen, touched, and so on, ICONOGRAPHIC, instead of merely phonetically alphabetic. This then gave them a further, wholly distinct set of determinative or descriptive media, which we lack in our Botany completely. We may *name* the plant, *describe* it in words, or draw its *picture,* just as Hernández did in his great volume, and we still today; the Mexicans did this also, but further added definitive written symbols, which then automatically fixed the Classes, Orders, Families and Genera as set forth in our here preceding pages.

To show these figures we have the wholly invaluable Codex Mendoza, covering pre-Conquest life and affairs, and including nearly 400 place names that incorporate the above symbols, from which (with a few from minor sources) we draw the illustrations here following. In doing this we shall roughly follow the divisions they made of the plant world, beginning with the trees; the place name is first given, separated by hyphens the better to show the reader the etymological construction and meanings, then the English translation, and with a few of our own defined botanical terms. To the thirty-three iconographic figures from the Mendoza, five pictorial ones are added from Sahagún's work, in complement.

The first of the little etchings shown in the margin thus gives us the name of the town *Cuauhyo-can,* or the place of many trees, or of the dense woods. Here the usual 'mountain' sign stands for 'place,' and on it we see the characteristic glyph for a tree, the brown woody trunk and limbs and three topping green ends to represent the 'herbaceous' part, the leaves.

Next we have a dwarf oak, Quercus parva, for the town *Ahua-tzitzin-co,* among the small oaks. The brown and green trunk and leaves, with the blue flowing water sign added; only part of the main trunk is shown, to denote the *tzitzin,* 'small,' and this reinforced by the regular glyph for something half-sized, the lower half of a human body. Another similar place-name, that for *Ahua-tepec*, is shown by the usual grassy green mountain, topped by the full tree, with the limbs, branches and water tips.

Our third town name, *Oco-a-pan*, is described on page ix, with its brown trunk, conoid inflorescence, green branches and yellow needle tips, cuts to draw out the resin from the trunk, and with water flowing in the bend of the green banks.

The cypress was the chief wood used for musical instruments, especially the great *teponaztlis* or drums; as such the tree itself was the 'drum-wood,' or waterside tree, the *a-huehuetl,* from which we then get the name *A-huehue-pan*, place of the cypress trees, showing the tree above a drum.

The town *Mizqui-c* had its name all written out as being the house or home of the mesquites, Prosopis dulcis; we see the known sign for a house, the reddish spiny stalks, the green leaves and the red and yellow legumes or pods, typical of the Leguminosae. This tree yields a gum like the Senegal, at times used in making ink.

Another 'place of many mesquite trees' had its name and that of the tree shown as here in the margin; we see the same red and white spiny trunk, the branches and pods as before, and below the trunk red rootlets instead of the other and differently shaped and colored plant bases, for water, stones, the bulbous root of the potato, and the rest, and as named in the above discussed terminology. This is the town *Mizqui-tlan.*

Other legume bearing trees, the mimosas, the Acacia albicans, we find growing around the town *Huizach-ti-tlan,* the 'place of many mimosas.' A similar root base, white trunk and branches with red spines, green leaves and drooping, curving yellow pods. The ending *-tlan,* instead of *-pan,* is here as often shown by the double row of teeth beside the trunk; why the glyph has this form is not clear, but the use is constant and definite.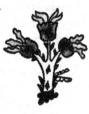

— xxxix —

Xochi-cuauh-ti-tlan, ' flower-tree-at-place,' took its fame and name, and doubtless also its main livelihood, from its many *xochi-ocotzotl* 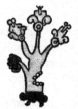 balsam trees, as to which see under the word *Ocotl, ocot-zotl* in the final index, and also the town name *Oxi-tlan,* below. The balsam in question was said to have been invented by the goddess of Medicine herself, and based on the turpentine exudations of the Pine. Perhaps the same as known as liquid-ambar, styraflua. The root is red, trunk brown, one branch at the side with the usual green leaves, the three main upper ones bearing the typical yellow flowers; the ' teeth ' place sign at the side.

The ends of the willow branches vary, as here seen branching separately and not in solid bodies; otherwise the tree is drawn and colored as usual. It also stands in the midst of flowing water, and the whole gives us the road sign of *A-huexoyo-can,* or the place of the willows.

Next we come to *Teo-noch-ti-tlan,* the place of the divine, the gods' cactus; below we see half of the sun sign, in red, green and yellow; above the three green cactus stalks, with their red spines, and the blossom topping the center, white, red and yellow. A pictured *teo-nochtli* is also shown on page 28 of our present Herbal.

From trees and cacti we next come to the Families of fruits and their trees; first the sweet in taste, with the zapotes as the genus type. For these plum-like fruits, our Casimiroa edulis, we can first take the town of *Tzapo-tlan,* its glyph the maximum of simplicity: red roots and all the rest of the plant green, including the round ends typifying the fruit itself; the ' teeth ' place-sign condensed, and set on the trunk.

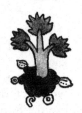

At the town of *Xoco-noch-co* we shall find ourselves at the place where are to be found the bitter cactus or tunas. Again we see the red root, three green stalks with the many red spines, and each of the three topped by the same flowers. The place name here is also of that north-west province of Guatemala, as now corrupted to Soco-nusco.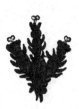

 Again we have a zapote species in the *te-* or *tetzon-tzapotes* or mameys. The town is *Tzon-tzapotla,* and seems also to have been known as *Toto-tlan,* place of birds, as see the bird's head incorporated in the glyph. Below, in place of the red root, we see the bi-colored stone sign, for the *te-;* then the bird, above the brown woody trunk and branches, then the leaves and fruit all green.

At *Te-tzapo-ti-tlan* we further have the town or place of the *tezon-tzapotls,* or stone-zapotes. We again have the bi-colored stone symbol, but it is more probable that in these two cases, as being fruit trees, the stone is indicative of the stony pit rather than a stony ground below. As before, and as becomes a fruit plant, stalk and the three branches are all green, while each branch bears two green fruits.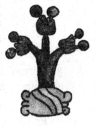

 For the coamitl, or wild blackberry, Spanish zarzamora, Rubus fructicosus, with edible berries, we see these here shown in a vase with feet, and a current of water running down past a *xomulli* or corner; this last, as also the bowl, is brown, either for wood or baked clay. The whole thus names for us the town of *Coa-xomul-co.*

At *Capul-a-pan* we find a much-colored glyph showing us a cherry tree, Cerasus capulin, growing in the blue waters of a channel. The brown trunk and branches, and green leaves are as usual, with branches of red cherries on green central stems, to complete the symbol. The town is also called *Capul-huac,* this term meaning ' cherried.'

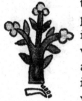

Passing on to the class of rather bitter fruits, of which the jocote is the genus type, we find the town of Xoco-yo-can, or the place with xocotl fruit trees. Here the color of the fruit itself changes to yellow. The trunk and branches brown, with green leaves springing directly from the woody parts, and three yellow fruit to each branch. The 'place' sign is also changed to that of a human footprint. The same yellow fruit reappear, this time from solid green trunk and branches, and the usual red root, in the glyph for Xoco-tla.

In this curious glyph for the town Ichca-atoya-c we see the sign for cotton, the plants apparently growing in a stream of water that flows out of a rocky place at the left, as shown by the usual bi-colored stone symbol. The cotton balls are pinkish, with a green peduncle. Similar cotton balls and peduncle appear also for the towns Ichca-teopan, 'cotton temple,' and Ichca-tlan, the cotton place.

After this we have the very simple sign for Me-tepec, maguey hill or mountain. The hill is green, as are the broad thick pencas of the plant. The root and penca tips are red, and the spiny edges clearly shown.

Ohua-pan means the place of many tender shoots of maize, or of many maize-sown fields. It shows the whole plant green, herbaceous, with uncolored roots, a red flower at the side, and long bending tops of yellow.

The glyph in the margin shows us 'burned over ground,' tlachinol-ti-c. We find the same term captioned at page 41 in our Herbal, where we are shown a 'plant growing in a burned-over place,' tlachinolpanixua-xihuitl. Here now we see a green hill, topped by what can perhaps stand for red flames over the dry yellow ground.

The cane plants we find everywhere growing, and which gave their name, Acatl, to the first day of the Mexican calendar, appear in no less than twelve place names in the Codex Mendoza, four of which are here shown. These are for the towns *Aca-miltzin-co*, cane in a small milpa or plantation; *Aca-tepec*, cane mountain; *Aca-t-icpac*, ' on top of a hill '; and *Aca-zaca-tla*, the place of cane and much grass. In

the first of these the small rectangle, marked in squares, and the ' half ' sign below, denotes the ' little milpa,' the green plant with red and yellow flowers the Cane. The next with its blue-green plant and cane glyph, on a mountain, explains itself. In the next the ending *-icpac* is the preposition ' above, on top of,' the hill below. The fourth shows two stalks of blue-leaved cane, in front of three stalks, or a quantity of fodder grass, colored yellow.

In *Teo-chia-pan*, place of the gods ' (or the divine) *chian*, we have below a dotted semicircle, which we are told is the symbol for the *chian*, surrounded by water, and above half of the Sun sign, which we saw above with the *Teo-nochtli*. The *chian* is a Labiada, classified as Salvia chian, for which see in the Plant Index at the end.

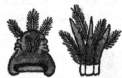 In *Zaca-tepec*, we have the mountain, hill or place covered with grass, and from the second sign in the margin we must understand *Zaca-tul-lan*, or the place of tule rushes turned dry or grasslike; although this latter value may be doubt-ful, the name meaning only place of rushes and grass.

This sign, with its name *Tolli-man*, is however not in doubt as to its meaning. The grasping hand stands equally for the *ma* of *matia*, to take, grasp, gather; hence we find ourselves in the place where they gather the rushes, the tule, that served the great industry of mat making.

Among the many kinds of thorns encountered in the plant world this must go specifically unidentified. The glyph means simply *Huitz-tlan*, or place of thorns. The body of the thorn is colored red, and the segments on the right blue, the same as on the glyph for *Huitznahuac* temple, where great festivals were celebrated at the New Year in honor of the god of war *Huitzilipochtli*.

From the place of thorns and blood-letting we must now seek the goddess and her place of healing ointments, the pine-drawn *ocotzotl* or *oxitl* above described. Its place, almost certainly that of its gathering and preparation, was *Oxi-tlan*. In a brown, baked clay bowl we see the black ointment, with a spoon or spatula, and above the white and red ' teeth and gums ' place glyph.

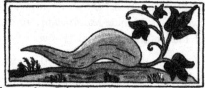

Among the roots of things we find two typical ones, that of the sweet potato, with its bulbous brown root and green herbaceous growing vine, shown here for the town of *Camo-tlan*, and below in a more elaborate pictorial drawing from Sahagún, of course in European style. Two other edible roots, from the Sahagún drawings, are also pictured below, one for the taper-formed root (again a generic class distinction) of the *cimatl*, harmful when eaten raw, but edible when cooked, as is graphically shown by the boiling pot and the youth eating the roots as they come out. In the Index is also shown the *xal-tomatl* plant, Saracha jaltomata, with its non-edible red tomato-like berries, and edible sand-growing roots.

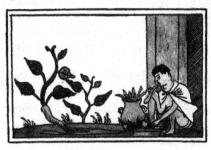

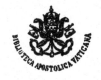

July 26, 1933.

Mr. William G a t e s
President of the Maya Society
The Johns Hopkins University
Baltimore, Maryland.

My dear Sir,

You will find here enclosed the last
aquarelles made by my niece, Marie-Thérèse Vuillemin.
Since the total of the flowers is 185, the total debt
is of Lit. 925 for the paintings only.

The photographs are sent under another cover
as printed matter, registered. The postal expenses
are of Lit. 21 for the preceding shipments and Lit.11,50
for these. In consequence your total debt is of Lit.
957,50, less Lit. 593,00 which were already received, i.e.
Lit. 364,50.

I hope the work will give a good result and
beg to tell me

Yours very sincerely,

(Mons. Eugene Tisserant)
Pro-Prefetto

-- 29 --

A LITTLE BOOK

of the medicinal herbs of the Indians, which a certain Indian of the College of Santa Cruz composed, taught by no formal reasonings but educated by experiments only. In the year of our Lord the Savior, 1552.

To the most eminent lord Francisco de Mendoza, the exalted son of the lord viceroy Antonio de Mendoza, the most illustrious superior of these Indies, Martín de la Cruz, his unworthy servitor, prays the greatest health and prosperity.

Since in thee the graces and ornaments of all the virtues shine, and those good gifts that are desired by any mortal, most magnificent lord, I in truth know not what in thee I may most praise. Indeed I do not see by what praises I may bring forth thy marked affection, with what words I may render thanks for thy exceeding beneficence. For thy father, a man most Christian and most devoted, I cannot find words to say how most of all he has favored me; for whatever I am, whatever I possess and whatever name I have, I owe to him. Nothing equal to, nothing worthy can I find, for his beneficence. I can indeed render enormous thanks to my Maecenas, but can repay in the smallest degree. Wherefore, whatever I am, I offer myself, dedicate and consecrate myself to his service. Nor indeed to him alone, but also to thee, my most eminent lord, for the most sure sign and evidence of my singular affection.

For, as I suspect, it is for no other cause that this little book of herbs and medicaments is so urgently asked for by thee, than to commend the Indians, though so unworthy, to his royal Sacred Caesarean Catholic majesty. Would that we might make a book worthy the king's view, for this is certainly most unworthy of coming into the sight of so great majesty; but remember that we poor and unfortunate Indians are inferior to all mortals, and thus our insignificance and poverty implanted in us by nature, merit forbearance. Now therefore I pray, most magnificent Sir, that this little book which by every right I should have put in thy name, thou shalt in this spirit receive from the hand of thy servant, through which it is offered; or, what I should wonder not at, thou shouldst throw it away as it deserves. Farewell.

At Tlatelulco. In the year of the Savior our Lord, 1552.

Of thy Excellency the most devoted servant.

A Table of what is Contained Herein.

CHAPTER EIGHTH: Curation of the pubis and groin, stoppage of the urine, difficulty in passing, affections of the rectum, gout, pain in the knees, the knees beginning to contract, remedy for cracks coming in the soles of the feet, lesions in the feet, against fatigue, trees and flowers to relieve lassitude in the administrators of the affairs of the state and the public business.

CHAPTER NINTH: The remedy for black blood, fevers, haemorrhoids, rectal swellings, excessive heat, cuts on the body, ringworm and tetter, recurrent attacks of disease, skin eruptions, wounds, disease of the joints, itch, festering with worms, inflammations, difficult digestion, swelling in cut veins after phlebotomy, those struck by lightning.

CHAPTER TENTH: On the falling sickness or epilepsy, the remedy for fear or timidity, a mind unbalanced or stupid, for one vexed by a tornado or bad wind, warts, hircine odor of sick people, phthiriasis or lousy distemper, lice on the head, protection for a traveller crossing a river or water.

CHAPTER ELEVENTH: Remedies for recent parturition, the menses, lotion of the womb, childbirth, tubercles of the breast, medicine for increasing milk flow.

CHAPTER TWELFTH: On boys' skin eruptions, and when an infant refuses the breast because of some pain.

CHAPTER THIRTEENTH : Of certain signs of approaching death.

CHAPTER FIRST: On the curation of the head, boils,
scales or mange, coming out of the hair,
lesions or broken skull.

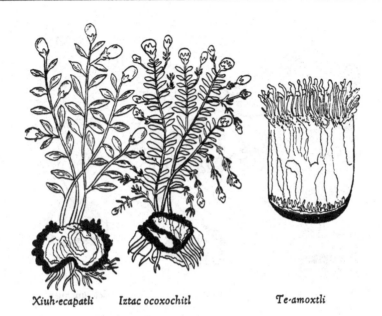

Xiuh-ecapatli   Iztac ocoxochitl   Te-amoxtli

Curation of the head

The fruit of the *eca-patli* plant, the *iztac oco-xochitl*, the *te-amoxtli*, the precious stones the *tetlahuitl, iztac tlalli, eztetl, te-mamatlatzin*, bruised up together in frigid water, allay heat in the head, and if in hot water an excess of cold. They are applied three times a day, morning, noon and evening, to be wrapped about the neck and throat over the supporting tendons and throat nerves. For pains in the head let him eat onions in honey, let him not sit in the sun, nor labor, nor enter the baths.   (a)

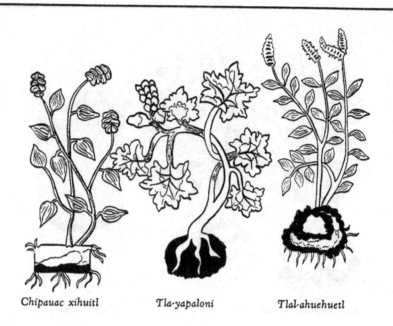

Chipauac xihuitl   Tla-yapaloni   Tlal-ahuehuetl

Boils

The leaves of the *tlatlanquaye* plant, root of the *tlal-ahue-huetl*, *tla-yapaloni* and *chipauac* plant, well macerated in the yolk of egg without water, will thoroughly cleanse out head boils; they are to be applied daily, morning, noon and evening, in doing which let the head be well covered. But if at any place the head is festered, it is to be washed with urine, and the ointment then used. **(b)**

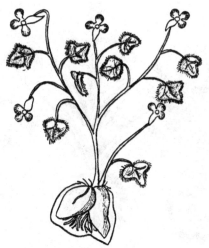

Quauhtla-xoxocoyolin

Scales or mange

A scaly head being diligently washed with heated lye, the juice of acid plants from the forests, well expressed and strained, is to be poured over the sores; when this has dried, the head scales are to be smeared with the gall of a dog, wolf, mole, hawk, swallow, the diver-bird, quail and *atzitzi-cuilotl,* with the dregs or lees of the Indian wine. As a drink let the one affected take heated native wine, to be drunk in honey that is not heated. Before dinner let him be very careful not to sleep, and after dinner let him not walk about, neither walk nor run, nor work. (c)

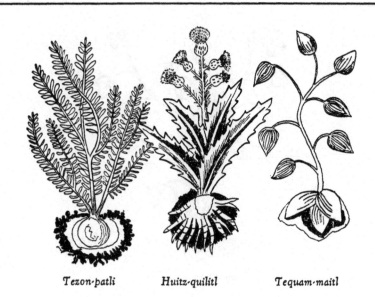

Tezon-patli   Huitz-quilitl   Tequam-maitl

Scurf or head-scald

The head is to be washed with urine. Then the roots of the *huitz-quilitl, tezon-patli, tequam-maitl, tetzmi-xochitl,* ground up with the bark of the *copal-quahuitl* and *atoya-xocotl,* are to be applied to the head. (d)

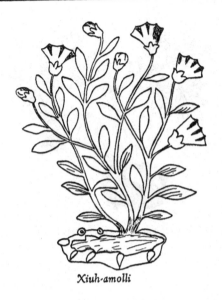

Xiuh-amolli

Coming out of the hair

Loss of the hair is to be stopped by a lotion of a dog's or deer's urine, with the plant called *xiuh-amolli* boiled with reeds and the *avat-tecolotl* animalcula. (e)

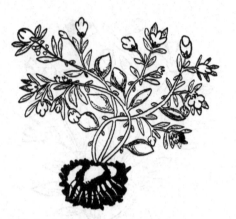

Xiuhuitl tonalco-mochiva hahauchcho

For a broken head

The break is to be smeared with plants growing in summer dew, with green-stone, pearls, crystal and the *tlacalhuatzin,* and with wormy earth, ground up in the blood from a bruised vein and the white of egg; if the blood cannot be had, burned frogs will take the place. (f)

CHAPTER SECOND: Curation of the eyes, heat, the eyes
bloodshot, cataract, stupor of the brows or rather lids,
tumors, to bring on sleep, to avoid sleepiness.

Curation of the eyes

If to the eyes, when in pain, one applies for a time white
frankincense and the dust of a powdered dead body, well
ground in dragon's blood and the white of egg, they will be
cured.   (a)

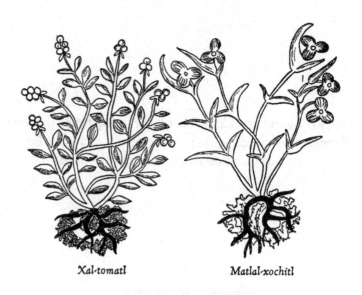

Xal-tomatl   *Matlal-xochitl*

Overheated eyes

Into eyes much heated from sickness the ground root of this bush is instilled; let the face be further wiped with the squeezed juice of the bushes *oco-xochitl, huacal-xochitl, matlal-xochitl* and *tlaco-izqui-xochitl*. Slightly troubled eyes are helped by the leaves of the *mizquitl* tree and of the *xoxouhqui matlal-xochitl*, macerated in woman's milk, or dew, or limpid water, and instilled. (b)

One suffering from a defect of the eyes should abstain from sexual acts, the heat of the sun, smoke and wind, not use *chil-molli* as a sauce in his food, not eat hot foods. On his neck he must carry a red crystal, and not look at white things but black.

The eye of a fox will help vitiated eyes wonderfully, being bound on the upper arm. If the eyes are so hurt that they look pulled out, pearls, reddish crystal, red mussels, the stone found in the small bird called *molo-tototl*, the stone *tlacal-huatzin*, and the stone in the stomach of the Indian dove, ground up in goose's grease, woman's milk and spring water, should be taken; the juice thus prepared you shall instill into the effused eyes.

When then something falls into the eyes, so that they fester from it, there should be instilled liquor prepared from ground siliqua or pulse, salt and flour, in spring water. If however the trouble comes from chill, it will be corrected if reddish crystal be ground in Indian wine and the liquor dropped in the eyes.

Bloodshot eyes

This trouble is removed if the suffused eyes are sprinkled with powdered human excrement. Also by the same remedy ulcers on the eyes, white spots, blackness harming the eyes; the shell of a fresh egg with the yolk, pounded up and with ashes strained in pungent or acrid water, let stand for eight days and then instilled, is most efficacious. (c)

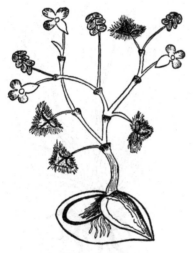

Ohua-xocoyolin

Cataract

A carbuncle growing in the eye should be lanced, then drawn and extracted; the film should be sprinkled little by little with the ashes from human ordure with salt. Then on the following day the roots of our acid plants, first placed in the sun, should be pounded up and applied. (d)

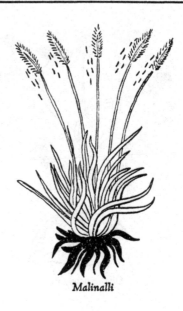

Malinalli

Immobility of the eyelids

When the lids are drawn with numbness, that is, when the upper does not drop and the lower raises but a little so as not to meet the upper, the leaves of the *malinalli* rubbed on the lids are useful; after this nitre, salt and powdered ordure should be sprinkled on them. (e)

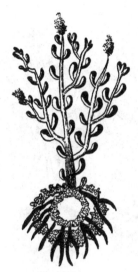
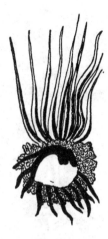

Tetzmitl   *Tequixqui-zacatl*

Tumors starting on the eyes

The bushes *tetzmitl* and *tequixqui-zacatl*, with the little stone, either white or the reddish, found in the stomach of the swallow, ground up in the swallow's blood, stops or restrains swelling of the eyes and a heat-inflamed face.   (f)

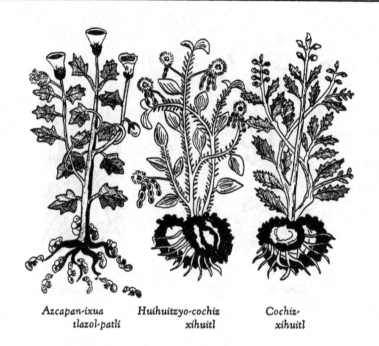

Azcapan-ixua   Huihuitzyo-cochiz   Cochiz-
tlazol-patli   xihuitl   xihuitl

Lost or broken sleep

Lost sleep is attracted and conciliated by the plant *tlazol-patli*, which grows by ants' nests; also the *cochiz-xihuitl* ground up with swallow's gall and applied to the forehead; also the liquor squeezed from the leaves of the *huihuitzyo-cochiz-xihuitl*, should be used to anoint the body.   **(g)**

To throw off sleepiness

You will drive off sleepiness if you will throw your own hairs on burning coals and smell the odor, while some of the incense reaches the ears. Not content with this, you may take a hare, draw and cut away the viscera, then cook it without water, to a crisp. When you have consumed it, take the ashes, to be drunk in moderation in water. (h)

CHAPTER THIRD: on festering in the ears, and deafness or stoppage.

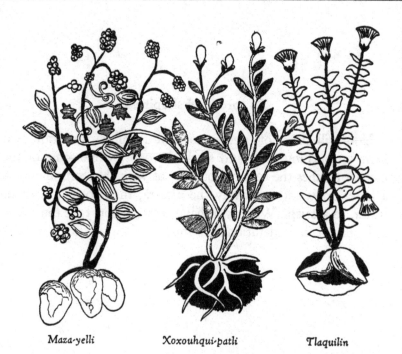

Maza-yelli   Xoxouhqui-patli   Tlaquilin

Festering in the ears will be helped the most by instilling the root of the *maza-yelli*, seeds of the *xoxouhqui-patli* plant, some leaves of the *tlaquilin* with a grain of salt in hot water. Also the leaves of two bushes, rubbed up, are to be smeared below the ears; these bushes are called *tolova* and *tlapatl;* also the precious stones *tetlahuitl, tlacalhuatzin, eztetl, xoxouhqui chalchihuitl,* with the leaves of the *tlatlanquaye* tree macerated in hot water, ground together and put in the stopped up ears, will open them.

CHAPTER FOURTH: on catarrh, medicine to be put into the nostrils, the blood-stanching plants.

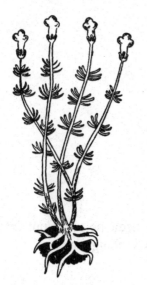

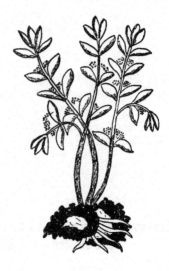

Tzonpilihuiz xihuitl   *A·tochi·etl*

Catarrh

One who has running at the nose or a cold will be helped by smelling the plants *a·toch·ietl* and *tzonpilihuiz·xihuitl,* and the catarrh thus cured.   (a)

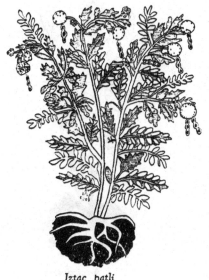

Iztac patli

Medicine to be put into the nostrils

The *iztac-patli* plant is to be crushed in a little clear water and the juice dropped into the nostrils of one suffering from headache. (b)

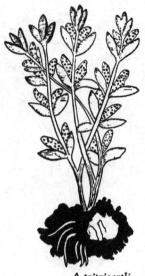

A-tzitzicaztli

Blood-stanching plants

For nose-bleed the juice of nettles crushed as a lotion, with milk, infused into the nostrils will stop it. (c)

CHAPTER FIFTH: tooth-polish, curation of swelling and
festering gums, aching and decaying teeth with much
heat, tumors and suppuration of the throat,
angina, medicine to ease pain in the
gullet, to bring back saliva when
dry, when the saliva comes
bloody, to allay a cough,
to stop foul and
offensive breath.

Tooth polish to shine the teeth

Rough teeth are to be diligently made smooth; the dirt being
removed, they are to be rubbed with white ashes in white
honey, using a small cloth, whereby elegant cleanness and real
brightness will stay.   (a)

Cure of festering or swelling gums

Pains of the teeth and gums are allayed by scarifying and
properly purifying the gums, while the seeds and root of the
nettle, rubbed up with yolk of egg and white honey, are applied
to the festered part.   (b)

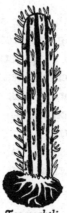

Teo-nochtli

Toothache

Weak and decaying teeth are first to be punctured by a dead tooth. Then the root of the tall plant *teo-nochtli* is to be ground up and burned with deer's horn; these precious stones *iztac-quetzaliztli, chichiltic tapachtli* and a little poorly ground farina should be heated with salt; all these wrapped in a cloth are to be compressed on the teeth for a while, especially on those where the injury or trouble with the pain is felt severely. Finally white frankincense and the kind of ointment we call *xochi-ocotzotl* are burnt over the coals, with the odor whereof a coarse pad of cotton is impregnated, and then is kept moving frequently between the cheeks, so as best to reach the pain spot. (c)

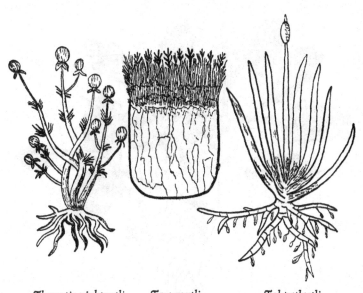

Tlanextia xiuhtontli   *Te-amoxtli*   *Tol-patlactli*

Overheated throat or pharynx

The leaves of the *te-amoxtli*, the *tlanexti*, with the root of the osiers called *tol-patlactli*, crushed in water, cool heat in the throat. With this is mixed the liquor of ground gold bronze or pyropus, and the stone *ez-tetl*, and then hold as much of this as can be, in the mouth inside the teeth, not passing it into the stomach. **(d)**

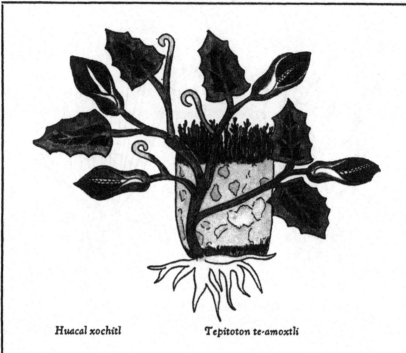

Huacal xochitl   *Tepitoton te-amoxtli*

Suppuration of roof of mouth and throat

Suppuration of the roof of the mouth and throat is cured by the root of the *xal-tomatl,* crushed together with the *te-amoxtli,* white earth, small or sharp variegated stones that are gathered from a torrent, *a-camallo-tetl,* with Indian spikes poorly ground, the flowers of the *huacal-xochitl* and *tlaco-izqui-xochitl,* of which the juice is well squeezed and promptly poured into the throat. (e)

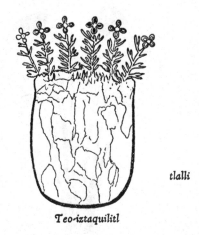

Chichiltic   tlalli

Teo-iztaquilitl

Medicine to ease pain in the throat

The liquor of the small herbs *tlanexti* and *teo-iztac-quilitl*, that grow in stony places, crushed in honey with red and white earth, reduces pain in the throat, if lightly rubbed on with a finger inserted into the mouth. (f)

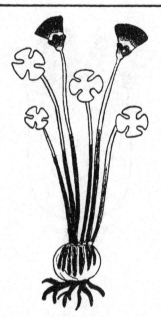

Quauhtla xoxocoyolin

Medicine to bring the saliva when dry

The saliva will flow and excessive thirst repressed if the acid herbs of the woodland, alectoria or the gems found in the maw of cocks, as also stated by Pliny, of crystalline appearance and the size of an Indian or Spanish bean, an Indian kite, a slain dove, are ground in clear water. Let one lacking saliva and immoderately thirsty swallow some of the liquor and hold as much as the mouth will contain. Also let the liquor of herbs macerated, the *tetzmi-nopalli* to-wit, and the *tepe chian*, be poured over the head; to avoid an error use the leaves only, not the plant itself. (g)

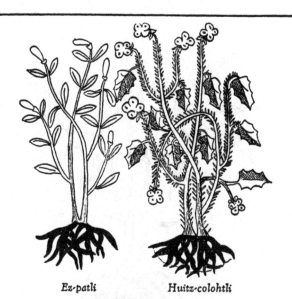

Ez-patli   *Huitz-colohtli*

For bloody saliva

For one spitting blood it is well to drink a potion made out of the root of the *tlaco-xilo-xochitl,* our pepper, the stones *teo-xihuitl* and *chichiltic tapachtli,* the bones of an ape, the red flinty stones you find on the bank of a river, white frankincense, the leaves of the *huitz-colotli* and the root of other plants whose tip is ruddy and small, crushing them in the whites of two eggs. Further to prepare the potion you should crush one root of the *tlaco-xilo-xochitl,* the leaves of the *huitz-colo-xochitl* and the root of another plant called *xiuhtontli,* the stone *teo-xihuitl* and the bone of an ape, burn pepper to ashes, crush together the *chichiltic tapachtli* and a stone found in the river, that is, in water; cook the bone in water with white frankincense, and then before a meal let him take one saucer of the potion thus prepared, for his drink. For one who spits out yellow mucus, take the *malinalli* plant, pine cypress and leaves of the plant *eca-patli,* squeezed in water or liquor containing ashes, or if it seems right in sour water; let the above be ground and cooked for a potion he is to drink; it is however to be diligently studied. This consumes the noxious humor. (h)

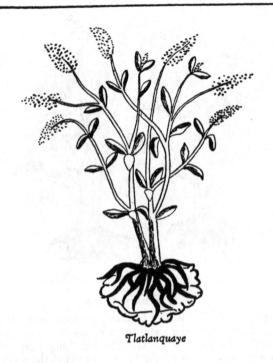

Tlatlanquaye

Medicine to take away foul and fetid breath

The root and leaves of the plant called *tlatlanquaye*, red earth, white earth, the plants *temamatlatzin* and *tlanextia xiuh-tontli*, ground and cooked in water with honey, suppress bad breath; the liquor, well strained, is further to be drunk before eating. (i)

CHAPTER SIXTH: for cooling the heat of a swollen jaw, to
cure one who cannot yawn for the pain, for scabs on
the face or mouth, for scrofulous eruptions on
the neck, dropsy, lameness or weakness
of the hands.

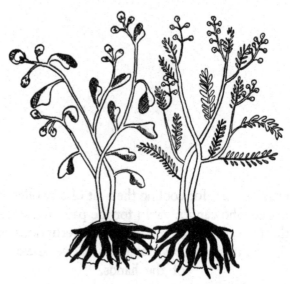

Papalo-quilitl   *Mexix-quilitl*

Against the hiccups

For the hiccups take the root of the bush *cohuatli*, leaves of the plant *mexix-quilitl*, bark of the red pine, leaves of the aromatic *tlatlanquaye* plant, grind them in water and boil them; when well boiled mix white honey and let him drink moderately. Throw white frankincense and *xochi-ocotzotl* on the coals, soaking a pad of cotton with the odor, and with which the chest is to be heated. Leaves of cypress also, with the herbs *papalo-quilitl* and *yyauhtli*, are to be macerated in water, with the heated liquor whereof the chest is to be rubbed. (a)

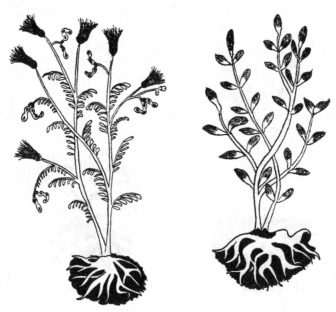

Tlaco-xilo xochitl   Tzopelicacococ

For a cough

If one is troubled by a cough, let him forthwith sip the boiled liquor of the *tlaco-xilo-xochitl* root skinned and ground up in water; using a part of this, with honey, to anoint the throat. If he spits blood also, let him take the same liquor as a drink before meals. It would help if he gnawed and chewed some of the said root, with honey. The root of the herb called *tzopelica-cococ*, ground in tepid water is also of value for one with a cough; let him either drink the liquor or gnaw the root. (b)

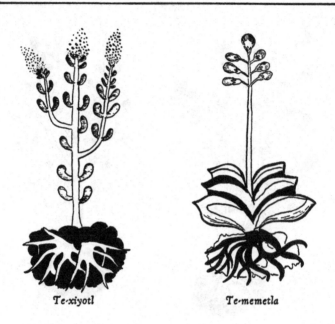

Te·xiyotl   Te·memetla

For swollen jaws

Swollen jaws are helped by taking in water the juice of crushed *tememetla* leaves, the pith of the *te·xiyotl* and white earth, the liquor whereof is sub-acid, with the gummy twigs bearing the glutinous tears we call *nocheztli*.   (c)

For those who cannot open the mouth the root of the *tlat· lacotic* crushed in tepid water helps greatly; if he drinks this liquor, making him promptly vomit, the freed mucus will open the mouth.

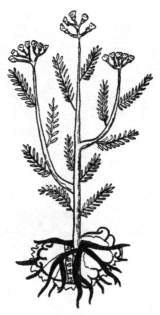

Tlal-quequetzal

For face scabs or freckles

To heal a scabby face, take the juice of crushed *tlal-quequet-zal, a-quahuitl* and *eca-patli* in water of an acid savor, adding pigeons' excrement, as a wash. (d)

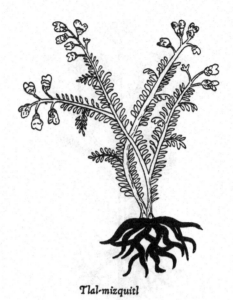

Tlal-mizquitl

For mouth sores

Scabs on the lips will be completely removed by a medicament made up of the *tlal-mizquitl* root, whose viscous drops or
tears are condensed to the thickness of gum, the leaves of the
eca-patli, nettle seeds, and pounded up leaves of the *te-tezhuatic*.

(e)

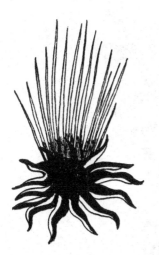 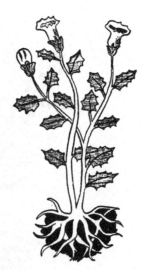

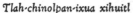

Tlah-chinolpan-ixua xihuitl   *Tolova xihuitl*

For scrofulous tumors

One scrofulous is relieved of the ailment if a plaster is applied to the neck, made of plants growing in a burned over
thicket of bushes or reeds, the *tolova-xihuitl,* the *tonatiuh yxiuh,*
the root of the *tecpatl,* and the leaves of bramble bushes; crush
these with the stone found in a swallow's stomach, with his
blood.   (f)

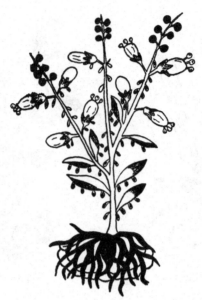

Tonatiuh yxiuh ahhuachcho

For glandular or spongy swellings

The tumors are to be cut with a small sword or knife, which done the matter is carefully cleared out, and a plaster applied to the cut. This then is to consist of the small plant *tonatiuh yxiuh* that grows in the summer, and *tolohua* leaves crushed in the yolk of an egg.   **(g)**

For dropsy

The water under the skin is to come out by cutting, and all purulence cleared out; this done, the leaves of bramble bushes and the *tzonpilihuiz-patli* are macerated and boiled in water with white frankincense, adding Indian wine. The medicine thus prepared is to be forthwith injected into the putrescent part, which is then covered up.   **(h)**

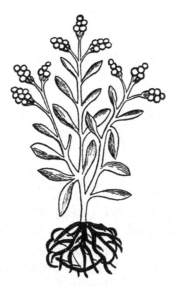

Quetzal xoxouca patli

For lameness of the hands

Lameness of the hands is helped by *xoxouhca patli* seeds, leaves of the *quetzal-xoxouhqui* and the herb *iztauh-yattl* crushed and boiled in water. In this liquor further the hands are to be put repeatedly and held a long while. After this bring on ants near whose nest a mouthful of meat or bread has been placed that they may congregate, and let him patiently allow the lame hands to be bitten by their mouth pincers. The hands are to be frequently soaked in the said liquor, and then wrapped in a napkin. (i)

CHAPTER SEVENTH: on chest trouble, pain in the heart
and heat, pain in the sides, medicine to kill worms and
animalcula, antidote for poison, tumor of the
stomach, pains in the abdomen, dysentery or
griping, rumbling of the abdomen,
chill, purging.

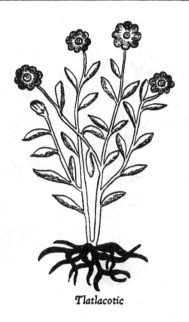

Tlatlacotic

For harassing stricture of the chest

When the chest is in some way constricted or drawn by any fulness, the root of the *tlatlacotic* is washed with hot water and then macerated. If so suffering pain, let him drink the juice in moderation; by this potion he will by vomiting get rid of what bound him. **(a)**

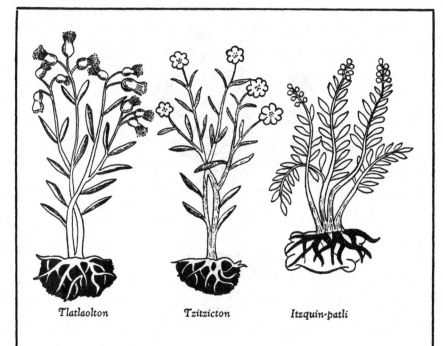

Tlatlaolton   *Tzitzicton*   *Itzquin-patli*

For pain in the chest

Pain in the chest is relieved by the plants *tetlahuitl* and *teo-iztaquilitl* growing on a rock, together with the stone *tlacal-huatzin*, and red and white earth triturated in water; the skin of a lion is also to be burned and its broth drunk; the chest is to be rubbed with the juice expressed from the herb *tzitzicton*, *tlatlaolton*, *ayauhtli*, cypress seeds or nuts, and the *itzcuinpatli* with the *huacal-xochitl* and *papalo-quilitl*. (b)

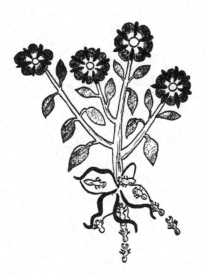

Nonochton azcapan-ixua

For pain at the heart

For him whose heart pains him or burns, take the plant *nonochton* that grows near an ants' nest, gold, electrum, *teo-xihuitl, chichiltic tapachtli* and *tetlahuitl,* with the burned heart of a deer, and grind them up together in water; let him drink the liquor. (c)

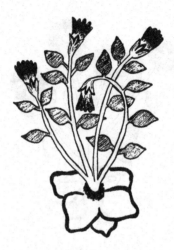

Tlaca-camotli

For burning at the heart

For heat at the heart take the juice from the root *tlaca-cam-otli*, white pearl, crystal, a very bright greenstone, beryl and the stone *xiuh-tomolli*, with *a-camallo-tetl* and sharp stones ground in water; this helps more. (d)

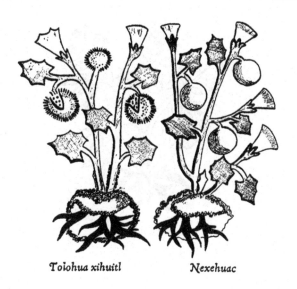

Tolohua xihuitl   *Nexehuac*

For pain in the side

For a pain in the side apply the plants called *tolohua-xihuitl* and *nexehuac*. (e)

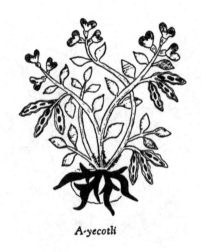

A-yecotli

Against animalcula that descend into a man's stomach

When one swallows animalcula, crush Indian beans and place in his mouth; then let him enter a well heated bath. When he feels the heat thoroughly, let him sip bitter water, without taking it down. Then if God wills he will eliminate the animalculum through the mouth by vomiting, or through the abdomen behind; or it may die there, and then when *it is* ejected, let him drink *tlatlanquaye* crushed in the finest Indian wine. (f)

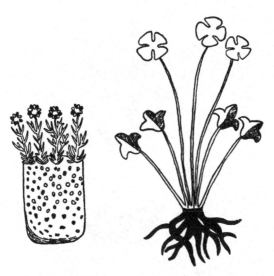

Teo-iztaquilitl   Tonatiuh yxiuh pepetlaca

Medicine to kill worms

Let the herbs *tzonpilihuiz-xihuitl* and *ahhuachcho tonatiuh-yxiuh* be ground with frankincense and boiled. Let the broth well cooked be clarified and then drunk, which will get rid of the worms.   (g)

Antidote

Against poison let a potion be taken prepared from the leaf and root of the *tonatiuh-yxiuh*, the root of the *teo-iztaquilitl*, the *xoxouhqui-itzli*, the *tonatiuh-yxiuh ahhuachcho*, ground together in water, with which are also to be ground up the bright pearl, sardonyx and *xiuh-tomolli*.   (h)

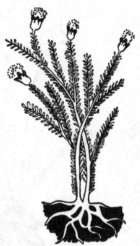

Copaliyac xiuhtontli

Tumor of the stomach

For a tumor of the abdomen or stomach, make a preparation from the leaves of the *xiuhtontli* and the root of the *tlatlanquaye*, the *copaliyac-xiuhtontli* and the alectorium or gem found in the maw of a cock, ground together in the finest Indian wine; also let him be given through the rectum a purge for the bowel made from the root of the *cococ-xiuhuitl*, Indian pepper, salt, nitre and the alectorium.   (i)

Pain in the belly

Let the root of the plant *ohua-xocoyolin* and alectorium be ground together, and the liquor to be taken into the abdomen by the posterior part; as a drink also give him the ground root of the plant *huitz-mallotic*.   (j)

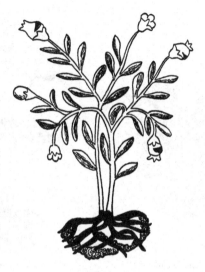

Xa-xocotl

Dysentery

The following serve well against dysentery: leaves of the herb *tlacomatl*, leaves of the *xa-xocotl*, almonds, laurel, almond husks, pine bark, the *quetzal-ylin*, the *ylin*, *capul-xihuitl* and alectorium, deer's horn burned to ashes, greens and grain ground up in hot water. The liquor is then to be taken into the rear parts by injection. (k)

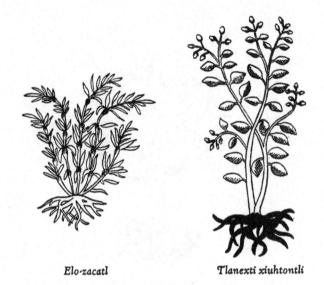

Elo-zacatl   *Tlanexti xiuhtontli*

For a rumbling in the abdomen

For one whose intestines rumble because of some flux in the abdomen, let him take by means of an ear syringe (clyster oriculario), a liquor prepared from leaves of the *tlatlanquaye* herb, the bark of the *quetzal-ylin, iztac-oco-xochitl* leaves, and the herbs *tlanexti-xiuhtontli, elo-zacatl,* the tree *tlanextia-quahuitl,* ground up in acidulous water with ashes, a little honey, salt, pepper, alectorium and finally *pizietl* or tobacco.

(1)

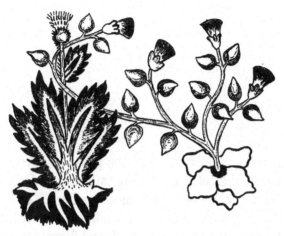

Quauhtla huitz-quilitl   *Huelic patli*

Abdominal chill

This is removed by taking a drink made of the roots of the plants *copaliyac-xiuhtontli, tlanexti-xiuhtontli, chichic-xihuitl* and the *quauhtla huitz-quilitl*, with added Indian wine.   (m)

Ventral purgation

When ventral pus forms, you will expel it if before meals the patient drinks a potion, in hot water, of the ground root of the plant called *huelic-patli;* the patient's bed, or where he lies, is to be impregnated with the odor of frankincense, whereby the noxious air is driven away.   (n)

CHAPTER EIGHTH: Curation of the pubis and groin, stoppage
of the urine, difficulty in passing, affections of the rectum,
gout, pain in the knees, the knees beginning to contract,
remedy for cracks coming in the soles of the feet, lesions
in the feet, against fatigue, trees and flowers to relieve
lassitude in the administrators of the affairs of the
state and the public business.

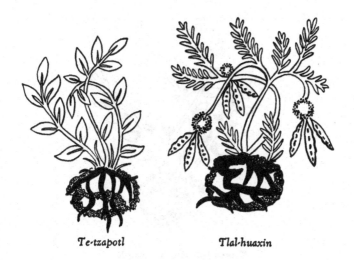

Te-tzapotl   Tlal-huaxin

Curation of the pubis

When this part feels pain, let it be anointed with liquor expressed and prepared from the bark and leaves of the tree *macpal-xochitl*, the thorny plants *tolohua-xihuitl* and *xiuh-tontli*, Indian knives, flints, the fruit we call *te-tzapotl* and the stone *te-xoxoctli*, ground up in the blood of a swallow, a lizard and a mouse. You must remember to heat this liquid. Also if a tumor or the pain burns severely, do not hesitate on section; the cut you must purify and anoint with a liquid drawn from the roots of the herb *tlal-huaxin*, ground up in yolk of egg.

(a)

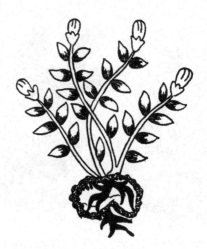

Tlanen-popoloua xiuhtontli

The argemon or groin plant

The plants *xiuhtontli tlanen-popoloua* and those that grow in a garden once burned over, the fruit *te-tzapotl,* brambles, *te-amoxtli,* the stone found in a swallow's stomach, ground in swallow's and mouse's blood, and applied, allay pains of the groin and reduce swellings. (b)

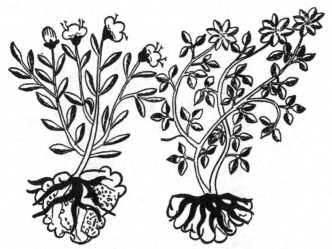

Huihuitz mallotic   *Coa-nenepilli*

The bladder-wort

When the flow of the urine is shut off, to open it take the roots of the plants *mamaxtla* and *cohuanene-pilli*, the *tlatlauh-qui amoxtli*, the very white flower *yollo-xochitl*, and the tail of a sucking puppy; grind these up in acrid tasting water, macer-ate the well-known *chian* seed therein, and administer it.   (c) The abdomen is also to be washed out with the root of the herb *ohua-xocoyolin* crushed in hot water, and the juice given through a clyster.   If this medicine avails nothing it will be necessary to take the pith of an extremely slender palm, cov-ered with thin cotton and smeared with honey and the crushed root of the herb *huihuitz-mallotic,* and this cautiously inserted into the virile member.   If this is done the stopped urine will be freed.

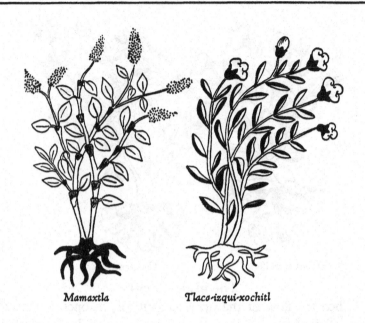

Mamaxtla   Tlaco-izqui-xochitl

Difficulty in passing the urine

Against difficulty in urination, a liquor prepared from the flowers *tetzmi-xochitl*, *tlaco-izqui-xochitl*, *yollo-xochitl*, the *mamaxtla* root, red earth and *eztetl*, white earth, drunk in water, will be of avail. Also place on the stomach a stone found in the stream, in which pearls (uniones) appear.　　(d)

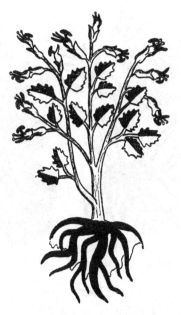

Coyo-xihuitl tlaztalehualtic

Affections of the rectum

Rectal affection is cured by the herbs *iztauh-yatl, tonatiuh-yxiuh, coyo-xihuitl tlaztalehualtic, iztac-oco-xochitl,* and the leaves of the herb *tepe-chian* ground together in hot water, with which remedy the part suffering pain is to be bathed; or they may also be poulticed, brought to mud thickness. **(e)**

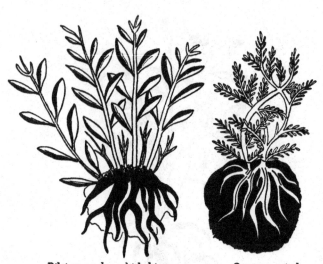

Pilzinte-couh xochitl chiyaua   *Quappo-quietl*

Gout

One with gout can be cured in this way: the bush *piltzin-tecouh-xochitl*, the leaves of the cypress and laurel, are thrown in an ants' ditch where ants go to and fro, or are sprinkled as a lotion. Then the leaves of the bush *quappo-quietl*, leaves and bark of the *ayauh-quahuitl*, leaves of the *quetzal-mizquitl*, *tlal-que quetzal* and *tepe-chian*, the flowers of any plant, a small white or red stone, the plant called *itzquin-patli*, pine, an oyster shell ground up in hare's blood, small foxes, serpentine rabbits (? for burrowing moles), *eca-cohuatl*, lizards; pearl, greenstone and bloodstone are to be ground up in water. If the foot is troubled with much heat, let it be soaked in the cold liquor; if it is chilled over the instep, it is to be heated. To the above named you also add a yellow-colored flint, and the flesh and excrement of a fox, which you must burn to a crisp.   (f)

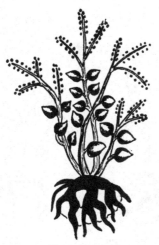

Xoxouhca patli

Pain in the knees

When the knees pain one, anoint them with the liquor of the plants *coyo-xihuitl, tepe-chian, xoxouhca-patli* macerated with the *te-amoxtli* in swallow's blood. **(g)**

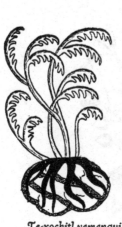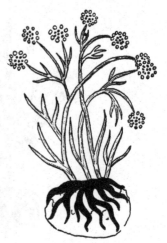

Te-xochitl yamanqui   Tzizicton

Incipient contraction of the knees

When the knees start to contract, anoint them with the juice of the plants *xiuhtontli* or *tzitzicton, yamanqui te-xochitl,* crushed in hawk's blood and that of a bird called *huacton.* Let the patient also enter the bath, and eat the cooked feet of the hawk, the *huachtli,* rabbit and hare. After that let the flesh of a very combative cock be boiled, which he shall eat, with some of it crushed as an ointment with goose grease. Let him abstain from sex converse, not avoid sleep, sleep sitting or supine, labor much, and not over-eat.   (h)

Cracks in the soles of the feet

Cracks in the soles of the feet are cured by a salve prepared from the herb *tolohua-xihuitl,* blood of a cock, resin, the resinous humor we call *hoxitl,* the which must be heated.   (i)

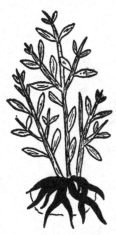

Xiu-eca-patli

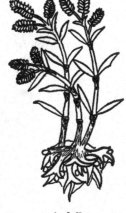

A-chilli

Lesions in the feet

For cut feet prepare these herbs: *tlal-ecapatli, coyo-xihuitl, iztauh-yatl, tepe-chian, a-chilli, xiuh-ecapatli, quauh-yyauhtli, quetzal-xoxouhca-patli, tzotzotlani,* the flower of the *cacaua-xochitl* and the *piltzin-tecouh-xochitl,* with the leaves of the *eca-patli* and the *itzcuin-patli,* the stones *tlacal-huatzin, eztetl* and *tetlahuitl,* pale colored earth. Then divide all this into three parts. Put some in a basin over the coals or fire that it may heat, in water, and put the feet into the hot water in the basin. Let the fire placed at the feet lower somewhat, that it may not fall onto them; the feet are to be wrapped in a cloth. The following day put our ointment called *xochi-ocotzotl,* with white frankincense, into the fire, that the feet may improve by the odor and the heat; also let the seeds of the herb called *xe-xihuitl* be ground up and put pulverized into hot water to apply to the feet. Third, apply the herb *tolohua-xihuitl* and brambles ground up in hot water. (j)

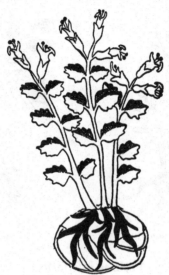

Huitzihtzil xochitl

Against lassitude

One fatigued will be restored if the feet be bathed in choice liquor, with the *ahuiyac-xihuitl* or *tlatlanquaye, tlatlaolton, itzcuin-patli, xiuh-ecapatli, iztauh-yatl,* the *huitzihtzil-xochitl* flower, and the stones *tetlahuitl, tlacal-huatzin* and *eztetl,* to be crushed in hot water. **(k)**

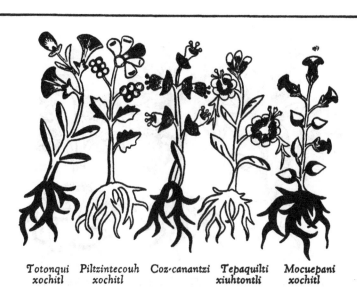

Totonqui   Piltzintecouh   Coz-canantzi   Tepaquilti   Mocuepani
xochitl   xochitl   xiuhtontli   xochitl

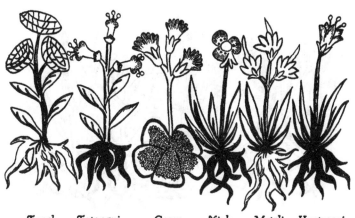

Tonal   Totonqui   Cecen   Xiuh   Metzli   Huetzcani
xochitl   xochitl   tlacol   pahtli   yzacauh   xochitl

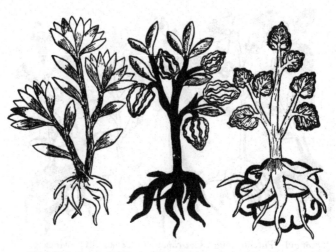

Temahuiztih quahuitl   Tlapol-cacauatl   Texcalama-coztli

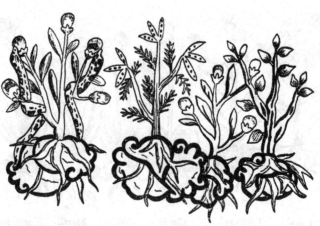

Coa-xocotl   Iztac quahuitl   Teo-ez-quahuitl   Huitz-quahuitl

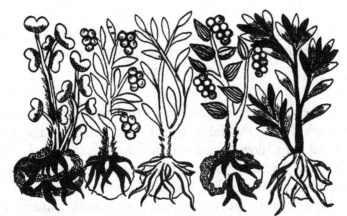

Tlah-cuilol quahuitl Tlanexti-quahuitl Te-papaquilti quahuitl
  Tomazqtl   Xococ quahuitl

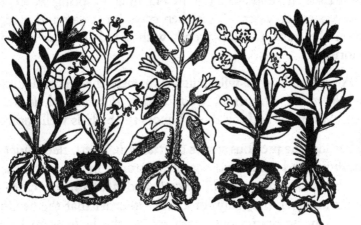

Temahuitztih quahuitl Elo-xochitl   Quetzal ylin
 Quauh-huitzihtzil xochitl Izqui-xochitl

The trees and flowers for relieving the fatigue of those administering the government, and discharging public offices

The bark of the tree *quetzal-ylin*, the flowers *elo-xochitl* and *izqui-xochitl*, the almond with its fruit, which is the *tlapal-cacahuatl*, the flowers *cacalo-xochitl*, *huacal-xochitl*, *meca-xochitl*, *huey-nacaztli*, and all fine smelling summer flowers; leaves of the trees *a-ylin*, *oyametl*, *ocotl*, *a-xocotl*, *eca-patli*, *tlaco-izqui-xochitl*, *quauh-yyauhtli*, *tomazquitl*, *ahuatl*, *tepe-ylin*, *ayauh-quahuitl*, and *te-papaquilti quahuitl*, flower bearing plants with their shrubbery, which you gather before the wind rises; these are expressed one by one in clear spring water, into new vessels or vases. This then stays for a day and a night, when the *huitz-quahuitl* wood, with a red juice, is added as coloring. (1)

Also the blood of wild animals, namely the red ocelot, *cuet-lachtli*, *miztli*, *ocotochtli*, white ocelot, *tlaco-ocelotl*, is sought for. With this and the above liquors the body is well anointed.

Second, the precious stones *quetzal-iztli*, *eztetl*, *tlacal-huatzin*, *tetlahuitl*, red earth and the small stones in the stomachs of the birds *huexo-canauhtli*, *huactli* and *apopotli* are cast into water in which they stay for a night in order that the healthful juice may be drawn out, with which the body is to be frequently bathed.

Third, the brain and gall of these animals, the red ocelot, white ocelot, *cuetlachtli, miztli, ocotochtli, coyotl,* also the brain, gall and bladder of the white *epatl,* ground up; with these the body is moistened. These medicaments healthily give gladiatorial strength to the body, drive fatigue far off, and also cast out timidity and strengthen the human heart.

As for the rest, let whoever wishes to follow through this reinvigoration of the body, eat other things also, but as of chief value the flesh of the white rabbit or white fox, either baked or boiled.

CHAPTER NINTH: the remedy for black blood, fevers, haemorrhoids, rectal swellings, excessive heat, cuts on the body, ringworm and tetter, recurrent attacks of disease, skin eruptions, wounds, disease of the joints, itch, festering with worms, inflammations, difficult digestion, swelling in cut veins after phlebotomy, those struck by lightning.

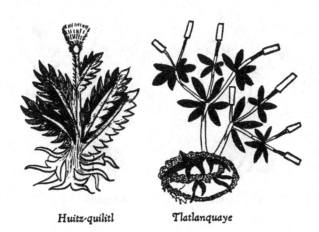

Huitz-quilitl   *Tlatlanquaye*

Remedy for black blood

The leaves and roots of the *quauhtla huitz-quilitl* and the *tlatlan-quaye,* ground up in water, are boiled, to them being added pearl, wolf's blood and our wine, which liquor thus pre-pared is to be drunk. Before meals let him at intervals drink the juice expressed from various sweet smelling flowers. Let him walk in shady places, keep from sexual acts, drink our wine in moderation, but only as medicine. Let him work at pleasant tasks, such as playing music, singing, playing the drums as in our dances. (a)

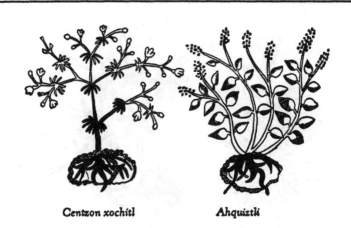

Centzon xochitl   Ahquiztli

Other plants are pictured above, which you may see in their places.

Fevers

The face in marking fevers has various changes, at times flushed, at times darkened, again blanched. He also spits blood, the body jerks and turns hither and thither, he sees little. At times bitterness, now burning, now sweetness of a kind fills the mouth, or rather palate. One who is such certain has his stomach corrupted. Although the urine is whitish, unless you avert the danger quickly the medicine will be prepared too late. Wherefore you will help him wonderfully if you macerate the plants *centzon-xochitl, teo-iztacuilitl, a-quiztli, tlanextia xihuitl, cuauhtla huitz-quilitl, tonatiuh yxiuh, tlazolco-zacatl, mamaxtla-nelhuatl, oco-xochitl, zaca-matlalin,* the bush *tlanextia quahuitl,* the stones you find in the stomachs of these birds: the *huitlalotl, huactli, aztatl, apopotli, tlacahuilotl, huexo-canauhtli, xiuh-quechol-tototl, tototl, tlapal-tototl, noch-tototl, acatzanatl, zolin;* the precious stones, fine green pearl, greenstone, sardonyx and *xiuh-tomolli,* with burned human bone, from all which a liquor is to be heated quickly and then drunk. This potion being prepared, the stone *texalli* is ground in water, and a part of the liquor poured on his head, his feet bathed with a part, and the throat moistened with part. Also let him drink some. Then these plants are to be crushed in bitter water, the *xiuh-ecapatli, tetzmitl, oco-xochitl, centzon-xochitl, tepe-chian, tzom-pachtin, iztac-oco-xochitl, tonatiuh yxiuh,* all of which are to be gathered in the fervent heat of the sun; then adding the willow and laurel and human bone, he is to be wet with their liquor. With this the tooth of a corpse is placed on the crown of the head. The plants *teco-xochiti—xihuitl* and *tlazol-patli* are crushed in woman's milk, and with this the occuput and nostrils are to be anointed; after all this is done, take heed that he smell a flower of some kind, and sleep during the day. (b)

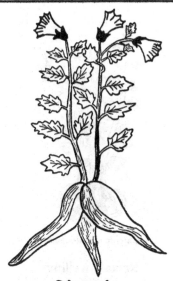

Colo-mecatl

Haemorrhoids

Against haemorrhoids the root of the herb *colo-mecatl* helps greatly, since it draws away the bile if it be drunk in hot water, crushed up with honey. Second, the plant *teo-amatl* that grows on the rocks must have the skin removed that the abundant milky juice may flow. Received then on cotton and put in the sun for a little while, it is to be drunk in moderation that the pale bile be drawn out. Then let a medicine be prepared from the skins of the plants *quauh-izqui-xochitl* and . . . . . . with salt, and ground in hot water; this will also draw the puru-lence from the abdomen and clear the intestines of the man. Before a meal let him kill a weasel and eat it quite alone with dragon's blood. (c)

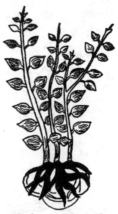

Chichic texcal-amatl

Rectal swellings

Oak-bark, that of the *huitz-quahuitl* and of the *capolla-xipe-hualli* and *tlaco-xilo-xochitl* are macerated. With these is mixed the *tlapal-achiyotl* and the salve called in our language the *holli*, the gall of a crow, root of the almond, bark of the *izqui-xochitl*, leaves and bark of the *texcal-amatl chichic*. A potion is prepared from salt, nitre and ashes, which is to be heated or rather boiled. Bread soaked with honey is brought gently touching the swelling. If this ailment starts at the buttocks, well heated water should be injected in the anus, and it should also be bathed in *teo-amatl* bark with honey. This then done, let the part affected by the swelling be frequently soaked with the juice of the *yamanqui-patli*. The *tlal-quequetzal* plant is to be crushed in hot water and the broth drunk.   **(d)**

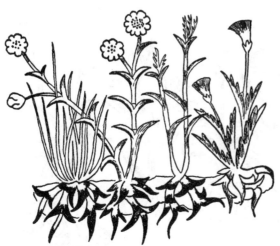

Acacapac quilitl   *Tzayanal quilitl*
        A-zaca-tzontli   *Acatl*

Excessive heat

The body when overheated is relieved by the ground roots of the *huitz-quilitl, xal-tomatl, tlaca-camotli, teo-iztaquilitl,* the stone *a-camollotetl,* the *eztetl, tlacal-huatzin,* red earth, white earth, and the stones found in the stomachs of a cock and the *noch-totl,* with sharp stones, all then put in water. This is drunk and the abdomen purged with a clyster. A potion is also prepared from *tzayanal-quilitl* roots, the *acacapac-quilitl, tol-patl-ctli,* the bushes *tetzmitl, iztauhyauh, huitz-quilitl,* with added salt. The body is anointed with the latex squeezed from the *acapac-quilitl, coyo-xihuitl, tlal-ecapatli, tonatiuh-yxiuh, iztac-oco-xochitl, centzon-oco-xochitl,* which are herbs; also using the leaves of the laurel, the bush *tetzmitl,* and the fruit trees *xa-xocotl,* the plant *cohua-xochitl,* leaves of the pine. This medicine is then divided, some poured on the head, some that is quite thick is applied as ointment on the body. If the heat rises, take the blood of the *huitzitzilin,* the gall of the *huexo-canauhtli,* the viscera of a quail, bladder of the *cocotli,* skin of the *pezotli,* burned together. These and the above are to be mixed together.   (e)

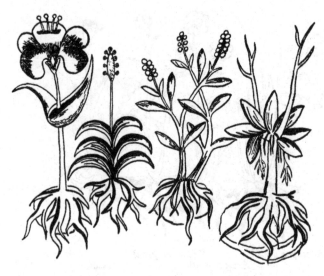

Tlazol-teo-zacatl Tla-yapaloni A-xocotl   Chicom-acatl

Remedy for lesions of the body

Lesions caused by rough treatment should be treated with a poultice made from *tlazo-teo-zacatl, centzon-xochitl, xiuh-tontli, a-xocotl, tlayapaloni, xiuhtontli,* moss from some tree, cypress nuts, seeds of the nettle, and the tree *ayauh-quahuitl.* Let the ill-treated one drink a broth carefully prepared from the root of the *coanenepilli, tlanextia xihuitl, chicom-acatl,* the flower of the *a-xocotl* and *izqui-xochitl, tetlahuital, eztetl, te-amoxtli,* the blood of an aquatic bird, the *huexo-canauhtli,* and some *tlatlanquaye* leaves, all of which are to be ground up in acidulous water. (f)

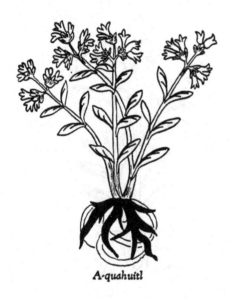

A-quahuitl

For ringworm and tetter

For one laboring with this scaly disease, let there be ground together and set over coals the bark of the cherry, of the incense-bearing *quauh-xiyotl* tree, the apple, the flowers of the *topozan* and *cacalo-xochitl*, oak roots, cypress nuts, leaves of the plants *tlatlanquaye*, *quauh-yayahual*, the herbs *tepe-chian*, *coyo-xihuitl*, *a-quahuitl*, cedar nuts and leaves; with these when heated let him bathe himself, and the affected part be rubbed with the burned pine, with which, and all the above, let him be rubbed.

(g)

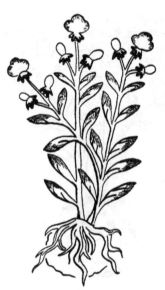

Cuecuetz pahtli

For recurrent disease

Let one relapsing in sickness drink, before a meal, a little of the latex like milk, expressed from the *teo-amatl,* that he may vomit. On the third or fourth day let him drink a potion formed from *tonatiuh-yxiuh* root, *tlatlanquaye* and also *tlanexti-yxiuh* root, ground up in tepid water. Third let him drink of the *cuecuetz-patli* root crushed in our wine. Let him drink this as he enters the bath, and then on coming out be anointed with the liquor of ground *teo-amatl* roots. The bowel should be twice cleared with a clyster, first with a liquor from *ohua-xocoyolin* root crushed in hot water, and this even though he partakes of some food; this healthful juice will throw out pus from the abdomen. The second time, a few days later, made of the intoxicating plant we call *piciyetl,* salt, our black pepper, and light colored pepper.   (h)

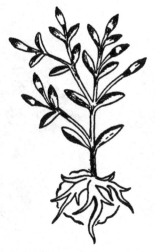

Ahhuiyac tlatlanquaye

Skin eruptions

The patient should first have the part affected bathed with urine; then let a plaster be applied made from *tlaquilin* shoots, *tlatlanquaye*, the *quetzal-ylin* tree, the bark and leaves of the *a-quahuitl* crushed in water. (i)

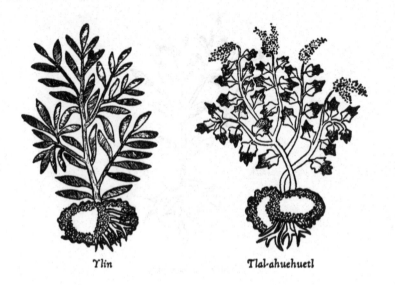

Ylin   Tlal-ahuehuetl

Wounds

An inflicted wound will heal if the juice from the bark of the *ylin tree*, the root of the *tlal-ahuehuetl* bush, wax salve and yolk of egg be injected. (j)

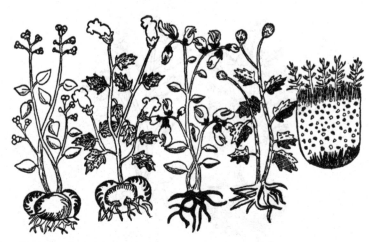

Quauh tzitzicaztli   Te tzitzicaztli   Patlahuac tzitzicaztli
                 Colo-tzitzicaztli   Xiuh-tlemaitl

Disease of the joints

Against articular pain, prepare a plaster from *quauh-tzitzicaztli, te-tzitzicaztli, colo-tzitzicaztli, patlahuac tzitzicaztli* and the *xiuh-tlemaitl,* which are herbs; also the many-footed serpentlike scorpion, all which are to be crushed in water and boiled. Further, a part with contracting stiffness is to be punctured with eagle's or lion's bone, and then anointed with the above plaster and honey. If the arthritic sufferer is moderately vexed by pain, it is necessary to puncture some part. (k)

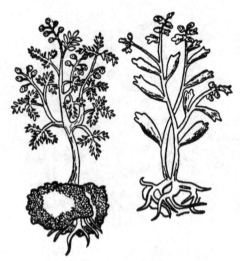

Tzihuac copalli   Tlaco-ecapahtli

Swelling of the veins after phlebotomy

When a vein comes to swelling after being cut, the bushes *tzihuac-copalli* and *tlaco-eca-patli, tetzmitl,* the root of the plant *tlanen-popoloa,* the leaves of the herb *quauh-yyauhtli* and *ahuiyac tlatlanquaye,* with the herb *coyo-xihuitl* are ground together with yolk of egg, in which water breathing the odor of frankincense is then poured, and the incised vein soaked with this liquor. (1)

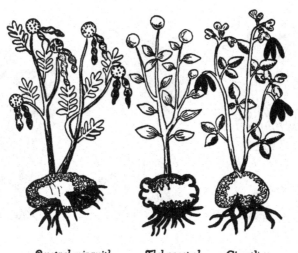

Quetzal mizquitl   *Tlal-cacapol*   *Cimatl*

Festered places with worms

When you see a festered spot gathering worms, grind together the leaves of the *quetzal-mizquitl, cimatl, tlal-cacapol* and bramble bushes; also the root of the *tlaquilin* and the bark of the *xilo-xochitl,* and put into our best wine; apply the liquor to the affected spot morning and evening. It will also be well to apply a medicament from bramble bushes, oak bark and leaves of the *quetzal-ylin, tlal-patli, quauh-patli,* and *tlatlan-quaye,* with the *tlal-ahuehuetl* root, ground up in water with yolk of egg. Use this twice daily, morning and evening, that purulence may dry up.   (m)

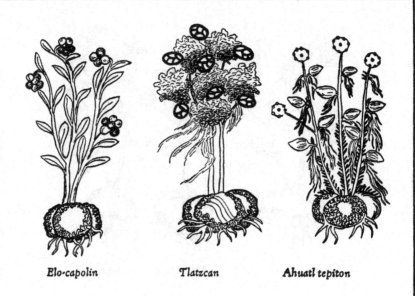

Elo-capolin   Tlatzcan   Ahuatl tepiton

Itch

When this roughness of the skin affects the body, use the bark of the trees cherry, oak, cypress, *tlanextia-quahuitl* and blackberry; also the roots of the plants *tla-yapaloni, tlal-ahue-huetl, tolohua-xihuitl;* the leaves of the oak-apple and the *tlat-lanquaye;* these are to be crushed, put in water with frankin-cense and yolk of egg, and boiled. The ulcerous or pustulent part is to be bathed with the lotion; afterwards the prepared medicament is to be applied.   (n)

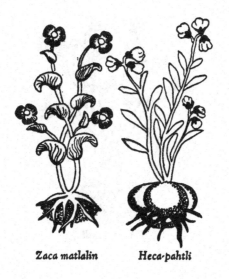

Zaca matlalin   Heca-pahtli

Dyspepsia, or difficult digestion

When any one by reason of overloading the stomach becomes constipated, give him cypress nuts, laurel leaves, the root
of the plant *zaca-matlalin,* the bark of the blackberry bush, the
cherry and the *ylin* tree, with the root of the *tonatiuh-yxiuh,*
which is red as bright gold. Then crushed together in acid
water let them be boiled with honey; the liquor drunk aids
wonderfully in clearing the bowels. (o)

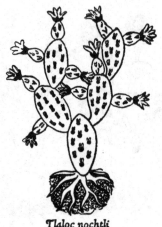

Tlaloc nochtli

Inflammations

An inflamed part of the body will be relieved by a liquor from the *nohpalli, te-amoxtli, tetzmitl, eca-patli, te-xiyotl* and *huitz-quilitl*, anointing the part thoroughly and rubbing it with honey and yolk of egg. **(p)**

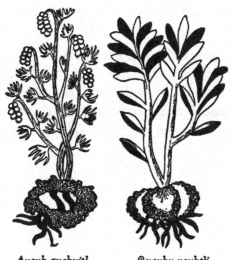

Ayauh quahuitl   *Quauhy-yauhtli*

Those struck by lightning

Let one struck by a thunderbolt drink a potion well prepared from leaves of trees, namely the *ayauh-quahuitl, tepaquilti quahuitl,* very green cypress, the bush *iztauh-yatl,* the herbs *quauh-yyauhtli* and *te-amoxtli.* But however the drink is to be given, let it be heated. (q)

Let the body also be anointed with a plaster made of the herbs *papalo-quilitl, tlal-ecapatli, quauh-yyauhtli, tlatlanquaye, huitbitzil xochitil, iztac-oco-xochitl,* and in addition all the plants upon which the lightning struck. A few days later let him drink water into which white frankincense is thrown. The water is boiled with white and whitish incense, with the burned bones of a fox added. Also mix some Indian wine with the above.

Afterwards you will instill into the nostrils a medicine made of white pearl, the root *tlatlacotic,* and all plants growing in a garden that has been burned over. Let also be suffumigated by white incense thrown upon the coals, the wax ointment we call *xochi-oco-tzotl,* and the good odor of the herb *quauh-yyauhtli.*

CHAPTER TENTH: on the falling sickness, or epilepsy, the remedy for fear or timidity, a mind unbalanced by a tornado or bad wind, warts, hircine armpit odor of sick people, phthirasis of lousy distemper, lice on the head, for a traveler crossing a river or water.

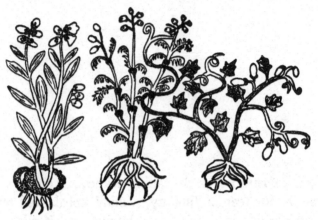

Quetzal-hatzonyatl   A-cocohtli   Te-tzitzilin

Epilepsy

Against this, recently aroused, there will serve the small stones found in a hawk's stomach, the bird *huactli* and the cock; with the root of the *quetzal-atzonyatl*, deer's horn, whitish and also white incense, the hair of a corpse, the incinerated flesh of a mole shut in a jar, all which are to be well ground up in hot water. Let the man affected drink the liquor that he may vomit, before which it should be well for him to drink of the crushed root of the bush called *tlatlacotic*. (a)

Observe the time when the epilepsy is to come on, for then the epileptic is to be instantly raised and the cartilage and sides punctured. Arising let him drink camnum gall, at the same time the head is given a poultice made of the *quetzal-atzo-yatl* and *te-tzilin* leaves, and the herb or bush *acoco-xihuitl*, all ground up in water. Let him eat the brain of a wolf and a weasel, boiled. Also fumigation with the odor of a mouse's nest consumed over the coals, whitish incense and the feathers of a vulture.

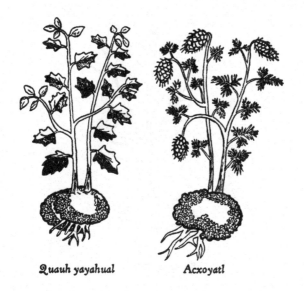

Quauh yayahual   Acxoyatl

The cure for one harassed by a tornado or evil wind

One who has been caught in a tornado, let him drink the
healthful liquor of the plant *quauh-yayahual*, the *acxoyatl*,
with pine and laurel leaves crushed in water. The broth should
be boiled and drunk thus. Drunk it expels the evil air entering within. Second: take the liquor of these stones, the red
crystal, white pearl, white earth, ground up in water, with the
leaves of the plant *tlatlanquaye*, boiling this with incense.
Anoint him with cypress and cedar nuts, and the leaves of the
plant *quauh-yyauhtli*, and those of the plant *xiuh-ecapatli*,
all ground in water with incense and the liquor carefully prepared. (b)

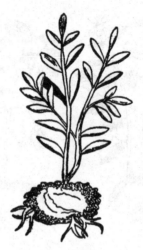

Tzotzoca xihuitl

For warts

One having these is cured if you apply the leaves of the verrucarium or wart-wort, macerated in water, to the warts, whereby they rot away. The warts will also be driven away by frequently washing them with water in which a human corpse has been bathed. **(c)**

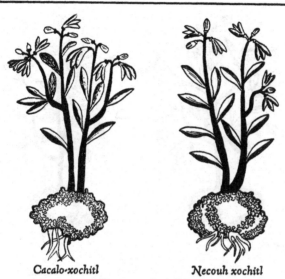

Cacalo-xochitl   Necouh xochitl

Fear or timidity

Let one who is fear-burdened take as a drink a potion made
of the herb *tonatiuh-yxiuh* which throws out the brightness of
gold, the herb *tlanextia-yxiuh, tetlahuitl* and white earth that
is to be sifted with river water; to these add the flowers *cacalo-
xochitl, cacaua-xochitl* and *tzacouh-xochitl;* he should also have
a poultice which you must prepare with the blood of a wolf
and a fox, a worm, the blood and excrement of the *acuecue-
yalotl*, laurel, swallow's excrement ground upon water, and
sea foam.   (d)

One frightened by a thunderbolt or lightning is to be anointed
by a liquor made from the struck tree, and the crushed leaves
and all plants which grew near the place. But let the water
used for sifting the unguent be of bitter flavor.

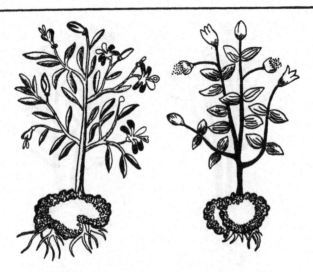

Cacaua xochitl   *Yollo-xochitl*

Against stupidity of mind

Let one who is possessed of such a mind drink the crushed roots of the *tlatlacotic* in hot water, that he may vomit. A few days later let the roots and flowers of the *yollo-xochitl* and *cacaua-xochitl* be crushed in water, and let him drink the liquor before eating, wherewith the evil humor in the chest will be largely driven out. Third: let the small stones in the stomachs of the birds *xiuhquechol-tototl* and *tlapa-tototl*, the *tetlahuitl*, the precious stones *tlacal-huatzin*, *eztetl* and pearl be ground together in water; after this divide the liquor into three parts, one of which he drinks and the second is at once poured on his head. Having done this, let him carry in his hands the stone found in the stomach of the *huactli* or night-owl together with its gall-bladder; with this and the drink he will come to himself and his sanity of mind be restored. Let his head also be anointed with the brain of a raven and a dove's feathers crushed and put in water with human hairs. On his neck let him carry the stone found in a swallow's stomach. **(e)**

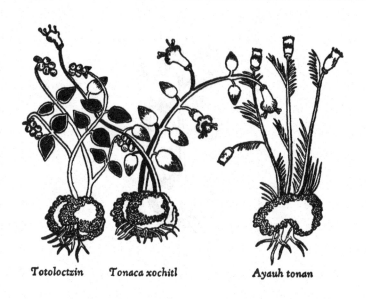

Totoloctzin   Tonaca xochitl   Ayauh tonan

Goaty armpits of sick people

This evil smell is removed by anointing the body with the liquor of the herbs *ayauh-tonan-yxiuh, papalo-quilitl, xiuh-ecapatli,* the leaves being macerated in water; also the leaves of the pine and the flowers *oco-xochitl, tonaca-xochitl, totoloct-zin and* sharp stones.   (f)

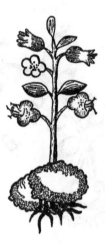

Chiyava-xihuitl

The goatlike smell of the armpits

When smelly and goaty, let him enter a very well prepared bath, and there wash the armpits thoroughly; coming out let him also bathe; for this take the crushed plants *chiyava-xihuitl*, a human and a dog's bone recently removed from the body, and the juice of all well smelling flowers and plants, with which the hircine odor will be dispelled. **(g)**

Lousy distemper

Numerous lice will not seek the body while one drinks a liquor derived from new deer's horn ground in our wine, or *octli*, of the best kind. It is also to be drunk frequently. (h)

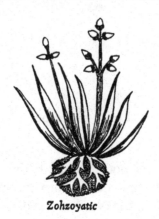

Zohzoyatic

Lice on the head

The medicament for this is the root of the bush *zozoyatic* ground in water of bitter taste, the herb *iztauhyatl,* the fat of a goose, the incinerated head of a mouse, the twigs removed from a swallow's nest, all which you must then triturate, and pour the medicament over the head.   (i)

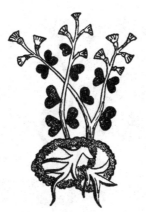

Tepe-papalo quilitl

Support for one crossing a stream or water

For one who wishes to cross a river or water safely, moisten his chest with the juice of the plants *yyauhtli* and *tepepapalo quilitl*, crushed in water. In his hand let him carry a beryl, the head and viscera of an oyster (?—sic), a sardonyx and the eyes of a large fish shut tight in his mouth.　　　(j)

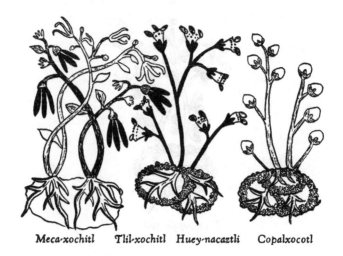

Meca-xochitl   Tlil-xochitl   Huey-nacaztli   Copalxocotl

The traveler's protection

The dried flowers *meca-xochitl, tlil-xochitl, huey-nacaztli,* the bark of the trees *copal-xocotl* and *atoya-xocotl,* the leaves of the *a-xocotl* tree, white incense, the salve *xochi-ocotzotl* and *yollo-xochitl,* thus crushed and pulverized; then crushed placed within the cavity of the well-known and most fragrant *huacal-xochitl* flower, that they may receive the very redolent odor of this flower, and breathe it out. Then take at the end the highly praised flower *yollo-xochitl,* which you must nicely hollow out and therein cover up the health bearing fine powder, suspending the capsule from the neck. **(k)**

CHAPTER ELEVENTH: remedies for recent parturition, the menses, lotion of the internal parts, childbirth, tuber-cles of the breast, medicine for increasing milk flow.

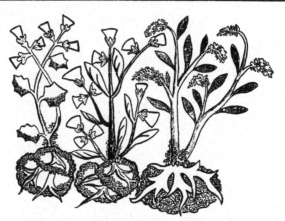

Quauh-alahuc   Cihua patli   Quetzal ahuexotl

For recent parturition

If the woman suffers difficulty in the bringing forth, then that she may give forth the foetus with little effort, let her drink medicines made from the bark of the tree *quauh-alahuac* and the plant *cihua-patli*, the small stone *eztetl*, and the tail of the small animal called *tlaquatzin*. Let her hold the plant *tlanextia* in her hand. Also the hairs and bone of an ape, the wings of an eagle, the tree *a-huexotl*, the skin of a deer, gall of a cock, also of a hare, and onions put in the sun are to be burned together; to these are to be added salt, the fruit we call *nochtli*, and the pulque we call *octli*. The above are to be heated and used for anointing. Let her eat the cooked flesh of a wolf, and greenstone together with bright green pearl be bound on her back. She may also drink the juice of ground up kite and goose flesh, and the tail of the *tlaquatzin*, in our sweet wine; also take the root of the *xal-tomatl*, the tail of the *tlaquatzin*, and leaves of the *cihua-patli*, grind them up, and wet the womb. Also grind the tail of a suckling *tlaquatzin* in water, with the plant *cihua-patli*, with which let the body be purged, it being given by a clyster.   **(a)**

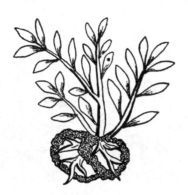

Hayuiyac xihuitl

Menstrual blood

The flow of blood is dried up and restricted by a poultice which you shall make of salt, ashes of a deer and a frog, white of egg, the hairs of a hare, the roots of the *ahuiyac-xihuitl* and willow, oak acorns and papyrus burned with deer's horn, the stone *eztetl,* pure gold, iron scrapings, all which are to be strained in river water, and the liquor infused where the flow of blood is heavy. Take and amputate the head of a lizard, extract the viscera and hang this in a cold place until it dries; then burn it, and let her be anointed with the ashes, mixed in Indian wine and white honey.   (b)

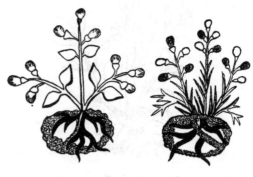

Xiuh-elo-quilitl　　　　*Tlaco-popotl*

Ventral lotion in childbirth

The womb of a woman entering childbirth is to be washed
out with the juice of the plants *xiuh-eloquilitl, tlaco-popotl,
centzon-xochitl, xiuhpatli,* laurel, all which triturate in spring
water with the stones *eztetl* and *tetlahuitl.* The feet are also
to be frequently washed with this. When the birth is about to
come, the *iztac huitz-quahuitl, malinalli,* white stone, white
nitre, pine, palm and *eztetl* are to be boiled in water.　　(c)

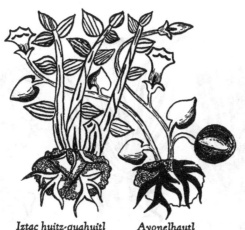

Iztac huitz-quahuitl   *Ayonelhautl*

Into the womb you also inject the triturated herb *ayo-nelhuatl*, eagle excrement, the acidulous plants, the root *quauh-alahuac* and the stone *eztetl*, that the pain may be lightened.

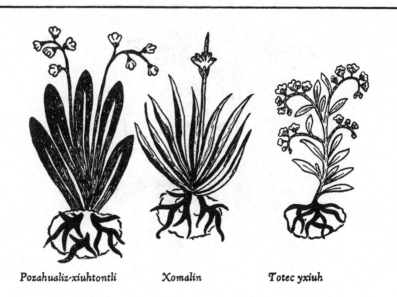

Pozahualiz-xiuhtontli   *Xomalin*   *Totec yxiuh*

Breast tubercles

For a tumor forming on the breast, take the ground up leaves and acorns of the cedar, leaves and root of the *quauh-yyauhtli,* the plants *elo-zacatl,* reeds, *pozahualiz-xiuhtontli* and *totec yxiuh,* and squeeze out the juice to rub on the swelling breasts.

(d)

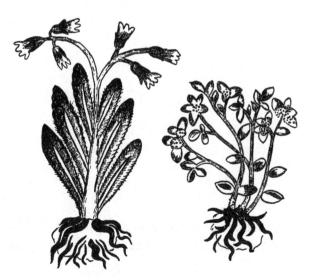

Tohmiyo xihuitl

Memeya xihuitl

To increase the flow of milk

Where the milk flows with difficulty, take the plants *chichil-*
tic xiuhtontli, which shows acid slightly, the *tohmiyo xihuitl*
and crystal, ground up in pulque and boiled Let her drink it
frequently. Afterwards macerate the plant *memeya xiuhtontil*
in pulque and let her also drink that juice; let her enter the bath
and there have another drink, made from corn. On leaving
it, let her take the viscous water drawn from the grain.   (e)

CHAPTER TWELFTH: on boys' skin eruptions, and when an infant refuses the breast because of some pain.

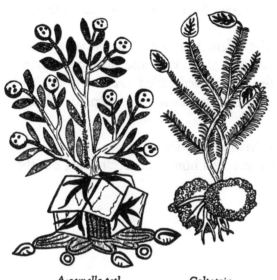

A-camallo tetl   Coltotzin

Infantile skin eruptions

Phthiriasis, or the skin breaking out on infants, is cured by anointing the body with a poultice made from the seeds of the well known *michi-huauhtli*, red incense, grain, which are to be burned; then the plant *tlatlanquaye,* leaves of the *huitzitzil-xochitl,* the root of the *tlal-ahuehuetl* and *tla-yapaloni,* laurel leaves, *xiuh-ecapatli* leaves from which the acid water is to be drawn; let the boy also drink medicine made from white earth, the small white stones gathered from the bottom in flowing water, the stone *a-camallo-tetl* and *coltotzin,* the bush *tlal-mizquitl,* and points ground in water.   (a)

When an infant because of some pain refuses the breast

When the infant is so affected that it spews out the milk and will not take the breast into his mouth, give him a drink made of the herb called called *te-amoxtli*, quail's blood set in the sun, and its hairs somewhat restored, which you will in-cinerate. (b)

Let him have a poultice carefully prepared from a weasel's brain and a scorched human bone, drawing out the acid water.

CHAPTER THIRTEENTH: of certain signs of approaching death.

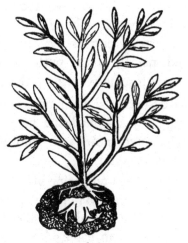

Quetzal ylin

The prudent physician will draw his auguries as to whether the patient is to die or get well, from the eyes and nose of the sick man. In his most likely opinion, ruddy eyes are without doubt the sign of life, pallid and whitish of uncertain health. A mark of death is a sootiness found in the middle of the eyes, the crown of the head growing cold and contracting into a depression, eyes growing dark and seeing little, the nose get-ting thin and pointed like a rod, the cheeks growing stiff and the tongue cold, the teeth powdering and rather dirty, and no longer able to move themselves and open. Also ever the grind-ing of the teeth, and the blood that comes from an incised vein either pale or else black, announces the coming of death.

Also the growing pale, or blackening, and putting on one or another visage, and finally the babbling of words without meaning or order, in the way of parrots. A special prognostic in a woman is observed, namely if the buttocks, calves and sides are as if punctured with some very sharp thorn.

In spite of this desperate state, it is still possible to instil into the dying man's eyes a medicine made of the precious stones *tlacal-huatzin, eztetl,* pearl and white pearl, with white earth ground together in water.

You may anoint the chest with pine wood crushed in water, laurel and the plant *tonatiuh yxiuh,* which you gather in the summer and keep for the occasion. Also puncture with a sharpened wolf's bone, or an eagle's bone, or that of a lion that is either white or spotted black in color, differently marked or sprinkled; to the nostrils you will hang the heart of an eagle covered or wrapped in deerskin.

At the extreme point, give a drink made of the precious stones the white pearl, the very green pearl, greenstone, whitish earth, the moss from woodland rocks, and *tlacal-huatzin,* which you grind up. Also from cypress nuts, which glow redly. Then the tree *quetzal-ylin,* the stones from the stomachs of the swift eagle, the quail, swallow, cock, diver-bird, *quechol-tototl, tlapal-tototl, noch-tototl, huitla-tototl* and pigeon, which you shall grind up together. Then indeed when the fatal necessity is at hand, and we are at change of death, the blood pours over the heart in a flood and spreading through all the members, death is complete.

Juan Badiano, interpreter to the honest reader,
salutation.

Whatever the work brought together by me in the translation, such as it is, of this little book of plants, most excellent
reader, again and again I beg that you will take with favor.
Truly I had much rather this my labor had perished, than go
under your most exact appraisement. You will further know
that I have put a number of hours in succession into this edition, not thereby to show off my skill, which almost is nothing,
but through the obedience which by highest right I owe to the
sanctuary of St. James the Apostle and Patron of the Spaniards, as to its priest and superior the very reverend Franciscan
father, friar Jacob de Grado, who laid this burden on my shoulders. Farewell in the Savior Christ. At Tlatilulco in the
College of the Holy Cross, on feast day of St. Mary Magdalen,
in the year of the redemption of the world, the fifteen hundred
and fifty second.

The end of this little herbal book, to which
Juan Badiano gave Latinity, Indian by
nativity, a Xuchimilcan by country, teacher in the said
College.

Glory be to him by whose grace I translated the book which
you behold, good friend reader.

Preface to the Analytical Index

The original manuscript of our Herbal contains 63 folios, three of which being entirely blank have not been included in the pagination. The arrangement of the text is in the usual form, *de capite ad calcem*, in thirteen chapters, with remedies for 101 ailments, usually one only to a page. There are 185 pictures of plants, and a number of others mentioned in the text, but not pictured. To avoid confusion, the pictures and text not always coinciding, the pictures are referred to by the pages on which they are found, always with an asterisk: as *ezpatli*, *p. 33, while all references to plants just mentioned in the text read, *Malinalli*, 3h, meaning section h of cap. 3; this also found on page 33, with nine other plants, though not pictured, nor is the *Ezpatli* above mentioned in the text below.

The Aztec names are hyphenated throughout, to show their etymological parts, with the meanings there involved; this is of the greatest importance for the reader to follow, and also because with the sharply integrated word formation of the often very long Aztec words, the whole meaning is dependent on such hyphenation. Thus since *a-* is the stem of *atl*, water, and *aca-* of *acatl*, cane, if we should write *aca-mallo-tetl*, a cane would be understood, whereas writing *a-camallo-tetl*, it means that the stone, or *lapis*, is held down, imprisoned "in the water," of course by the plants shown grasping it in the picture. Hyphenating the words, and correctly, is a simple necessity.

In this situation, further burdened by the great inattention to the keys of pharmacology and the absolutely essential real knowledge of Aztec as the language, we have in our Introduction and the following Index sought just to do two things: invite further study by others on these lines, and at the same time tell the general reader, as our space permits, what we can of interest about the plants themselves as a part of the pre-conquest Mexican life. We have ourselves in the progress of preparing the work for publication, learned much from the plant skill shown by De la Cruz, and his informative colored pictures of the plants he so clearly knew.

In Parts One and Three hereof we have thus tried to open the door to interest and understanding; we hope our readers will give their proper heed to De la Cruz and Badiano, and see through them, and once more through El Proto-Mèdico Francisco Hernández, a great background of science.

Many of the plants are definitely botanically, with our known terms; the ancient names of many have been lost in use, and the plant knowledge of even the 16th century with them. Long and intensive studies, from such skilled botanists as Sessé and Mociño, sent by Charles III to pick up and follow Hernández's work, down to Ramirez, Herrera and Alcocer and all the very capable moderns, have had to report this fact constantly.

In the Aztec words the *x* is to be pronounced *sh* (as it was in 16th century Spanish); *tz* and *tl* are treated as single letters like our *ch*, not to be separated. The accent regularly falls on the next to the last syllable.

Analytical Index to Plants named in Herbal.

Aca-capac-quilitl, pleasing cane edible. Aganippea dentata, *p. 79.
> Grows in the Canal de la Vega, near Mexico City. v. Sahagún, xi-7.8.20.

Acatl, cane. Arundo donax L. *p. 79.
> There are various reedlike plants, including edible ones, growing in or by water. Note the identical root forms on all four plants on p. 79, and also the similarity of the reedlike stalks for this and the next number.

A-chilli, water chile. *p. 65.
> While there is no actual identification of this with the Salvia chian from which was made the refreshing drink so universally had during Holy Week, yet our sources, taken in parallel, strongly suggest it. First, Sahagún, discussing the achilli at xi-7.5.86, speaks of " this chian "; further, the Madrid Hernández, i-270, speaks of the achilton, or small achilli, as having the synonym piltzin-tecouh-xochitl; and then, our present section of the Badiano prescribing a number of aromatics, gives us in succession wormwood, mountain chian and a-chilli, and just below piltzin-tecouh-xochitl.

Acocotli, or Acoco-xihuitl, aesophagus or ' suction pipe '; cumin. Arra-
cacia atropurpurea, *p. 94, 10a.
> The acocotli was used for sucking up the gathered juice of the maguey for making pulque, and the cane-like divisions of the stalk are plainly shown in the illustration. Three illustrations of an acocotli plant are given at Hern. 31, none resembling this in any way.
>
> Robelo quotes Molina as to the above use of the stalk, and then gives it as being cumin or Arracacia atropurpurea, followed here by the Ph. Mex. and then by Martínez, all giving it as stimulant and carminative, which the two paragraphs in Sahagún fairly support.

Acxoyatl, a balsam. Abies religiosa, *p. 95, 10b.
> The picture at Hern. 348 quite agrees with the one here in showing it as being of the Pine family.

Ahquiztli. Save for the picture at *p. 74, and its association with the
long list of plants prescribed for a fever, 9b, no guide at hand.

Ahuatl, oak. Quercus castanea L. Quercus insignis. 8-1.
> The Latin word Quercus is quite regularly used in the text, instead of the Aztec.
>
> We also have an Ahuatl-tepiton, small oak, at *p. 88, but not repeated in the text. At p. 211 Hernández illustrates the Ahuaton or Quercus parva, with the synonym Tlal-capulin; also Sahagún gives us these same synonyms, at xi-7.5.49; also the term ava-quavitl at xi-6.2.8; and at xi-6.2.8 ava-tetzmolli as the holm oak.

A-huehuetl, water-growing cypress. Cupressus Montezuma, or Taxodium mucronatum.

This also is only referred to by its Latin name, but its fame is such as to merit the following quotation from Standley:

"The largest individual reported is the famous one of Tule, near Oaxaca; its height is 38.6 meters and the girth 51.8 meters; the greatest trunk diameter is 12 meters, and the spread of the branches 51.8 meters. The Cypress of Moctezuma at Chapultepec was a noted tree four centuries ago, and its actual age estimated at 700 years; others have attained much greater periods.

"The tree has been long used for its acrid resin, curative of ulcers, toothache, gout; also as diuretic and resolutive and a pectoral."

Ahuiyac, adj. Agreeable; used with xihuitl, plant, 8k, *p. 107; also tlatlanquaye, pepper, *p. 73, *83.

Amatl, fig-tree; wood used for paper. Ficus nymphaefolia L.

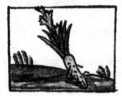

Xiuh-amolli, soap plant. Saponaria americana, *p. 11, 1e.

A small plant whose root yields a glutinous lather and supplies an excellent soap. Note the use of *xiuh-* as prefix, instead of a terminal *xihuitl*, to mark particularly its smallness and herbaceous character.

Amoxtli, paper plant or rush; also name for paper, book, etc.

We only have this as *te-amoxtli*, or a papyrus reed growing on stony ground; the illustrations at pp. 7, 29, and that of the small or *tepitonte-amoxtli* all show the marshy bottom. This marshy base is also seen with the *teo-iztaquilitl*, *p. 3, or Portulaca oleracea L, growing in "red earth," at 5f as growing in a stone-filled marsh. With these also note the marshy base of the *xiuh-tlemaitl* on p. 85. (See these latter in their places.) The *te-amoxtli* is prescribed seven times in the text passages, at 5d, 8b, 8f, 9f, 9p, 9q, 12b.

Paper made in ancient Mexico was of two kinds, one from the above papyrus, and the finer kind from the fig-tree, or Ficus petiolaris, illustrated by Hernández at p. 82 as the *tepe-amatl*, mountain fig, or *texcal-amatl*, rock-cavern fig. Specimens of this paper we still have in our few surviving codices, and it further gave its name to the sacred calendar-book the *Tonal-amatl*.

Sahagún tells us that the tree is of the size of a peach, its leaves very green, and the bark smooth; when this bark grows old, "they cut it off for the paper-making, whereon the tree puts on anew."

The wood is yellowish, whence the further term *amacoztic*. Its medicinal value is as a pectoral.

A-quahuitl, water-tree. Illustrated at *p. 81, and prescribed in the text at 6d, 9i.

> Not mentioned by Hernández, nor in our other sources at hand.

A-toch-ietl, literally ' water-growing rabbit bean.' *p. 24.

> Hern. 1790 ed., pp. 148-50, gives four species, all aromatic, and being the flea-bane, Pulegium, or similar. One of these is given as curing colds and headache. Apparently pennyroyal.

Atoya-xocotl, ' flowing-stream plum.' Spondias mombin L. 1d, 10k.

> Sahagún at xi-6.7.4 lists four plum or *jocote* varieties, calling them all *xoco-quahuitl*, or bitter tree; first are the yellow or red manzanillas, with white centers, called *te-xocotl*; then the *maza-xocotl*, or ' deer plums,' red or yellow; then the " large plum ciruelas called *atoya-xocotl*, sweet and savory, good to eat raw or cooked. They make a pulque of these that is more intoxicating than that from honey; all the plums have large pits." Finally the guavas, the *xal-xocotl* or ' sand-plums.'
>
> The modern Farm. Mex. assigns no medicinal value, but Hern., 1790 ed. iii, 355, gives a seven line paragraph describing the plum as being cooling, astringent, and of value in dysentery. The 1651 edition assigns the same qualities.

A-xocotl, ' water plum.' Spondias sp., *p. 80, 8-l, 10k. v. supra.

Ayauh-quahuitl, ' misty cloud tree.' ? Cupressus thurifera, *p. 91, 8b, 8f, 9f.

> Quite probably the white cedar, as given by Siméon Dict.; the trees of this family are usually called in the Badiano text by their Latin names, Pinus, Cupressus.

Ayauhtli, cloud or mist; probably the above. 7b.

Ayecotli, large beans, haricots. Phaseolus multiflorus L, *p. 50.

> Molina, Dict. gives it thus, as frijoles gordos; the term is immediately followed in the text as fabas indias, or Indian beans; next to maize they are the staple diet.

A-illin, water alder. Alnus acuminata H. B. K. Betula alnus L, 8-l.

> See also *Ylin*, 7k, *p. 84, 9o; *tepe-ylin*, 8k; *quetzal-ylin*, *p. 69, 8-l, 7k.

Ayo-nelhuatl, calabash root. Cucurbita maxima, *p. 109, 11c.

> The only time the Aztec word for ' root' is used instead of the Latin radix.

A-zaca-tzontli, ' water-hair-grass.' *p. 79.

> Pictured with three other water plants, but not mentioned in the text. Molina defines it as ' coarse hair grass,' *azacatl*, being given as paja gorda, coarse grass.

Azcapanixua-tlazol-patli, 'remedy growing in filth by an ants' nest,'
*p. 20.

The 'filth-medicine' is then given in the text with two other soporifics, and a swallow's gall rubbed on the forehead.

E

Just as the majority of our plants above have as their initial element the letter A-, the adjectival or prefix form of Atl, water, so under the E we have only three divisions, based on the words *Ecatl, Elotl* and *Eztli*, for Air or Wind, the ear of Corn or Maize when ripe, and Blood. Thus, however widely these terms or plants may be separated in our botanical classes, they should here be viewed and considered under these three heads, as did the native users who so named them.

While, then, the final element of each compound names the physical thing itself, as being tree, plant, flower, medicine or edible, the controlling descriptive part of the word is the initial qualifying and descriptive adjective (regularly dropping here the final -tl or -tli). This will bring the use-quality of each, always foremost in the Indian's mind, together and associated in their listing.

Considering the first of the three, the *Ecatl*, it should be noted in starting that it is very doubtful at the least, whether the Air was ever thought of by the Indian except as in motion, or otherwise *manifesting* itself to the senses. So far as our many dictionaries and texts show us, for all Middle America whether Mexican or Mayance, the air is an element merely, invisible, unfelt, unsmelt, or even untasted as in halitosis (see chap. 5, sec. i), is not to the Indian a 'thing,' and hence not of course a cause of trouble or disease. The universal belief in the 'bad winds' as causing misfortune or bodily ailments, is well known, everywhere; but this is always some maleficent 'influence,' like our 'evil eye,' or our present-day Pennsylvania 'hexing,' now so regarded as void of all foundation, but three hundred years ago the very opposite among our New England relatives.

Eca-patli, 'wind '-remedy. Cassia occidentalis L, Senna family. *p. 7,
*p. 65, 8j, 8k, 9b, 10b, 10f.

This we have as of two heights, the *ecapatli* or *xiuh-ecapatli*, mentioned 13 times, and with three illustrations, as above. Then the *tlaco-ecapatli*, the middle-sized, at page 86, this picture agreeing with that at p. 7, the first picture in our Herbal. Hern. i-265 also gives it as synonym for the low or *tlal-huaxin*, and one of the 33 varying kinds of the *huaxin*; he also calls it *totonca-xihuitl*, or hot medicine, also *xometontli* or small Sambucus, and again as *xio-patli*, or eruption remedy.

It has the same qualities as our Senna, belonging to the Senna family, and given as curing tumors, headaches, fevers and the spreading skin affection called 'lepra' or *xiotl*, which is definitely not the genuine leprosy, that came to the Americas at a now known date, after the Conquest. This is just as the Spanish word 'bubas' is persistently taken as standing for the technical syphilitic 'buboes,' in spite of the positive non-existence of that also, in America prior to the coming of the Europeans. Dr. Shattuck's recent work among the Mayas, under Carnegie auspices, definitely strengthens the early statements on this fact, while direct researches into early Mayan language sources have shown these so-called syphilitic 'bubas,' or *sob* in Maya, to be restricted to throat tumors, or scrofula, our 'King's evil.'

Standley gives us 24 species of the Caesalpinia or Senna, adding that C. tora has a great reputation in India, our antipodes, for ringworm, while from Oaxaca Dr. Reko cites C. alata as "*ecapatli*," a cure for ringworm. See further below under the *Huaxin*, the *huitz-quahuitl*, and the *xilo-xochitl*.

Elo-capolin, maize-ear cherry. Cerasus sp., *p. 88.

The text with the picture prescribes cherry bark, cortex cerasi, both for tetter and the itch, 9g, 9n, using the Latin instead of the Aztec terms.

Elo-xochitl, maize-ear flower. Magnolia aculbata, *p. 69, 8-l.

The flowers, like the *yollo-xochitl* or heart-flower, and others, were added as flavoring to the chocolate.

Xiuh-elo-quilitl, maize-ear edible. *p. 108, 11c.

Hern., ii-283 ff., describes one plant with this name, and six others as like it, *eloquiltic*, all being dry and heating, and one even with the pepper *tlatlan-quaye* as its synonym. But no further exact identification is found.

Elo-zacatl, maize-ear grass. *p. 54, 7-l, 11d.

On this Sahagún tells us that it is very green and soft, has heads like wheat, and is eaten by rabbits and other animals.

Ez-patli, blood medicine, 'dragon's blood.' Croton draco, *p. 33.

Ez-quahuitl, 'blood tree.' Jatropha spathulata.

Teo-ezquahuitl, sacred blood tree. Jatropha sp., *p. 68.

There is great confusion among all the writers as to this quite famous medicine. The first term above simply calls it a blood medicine, although Hernández clearly describes it as a plant, while distinguishing the two names, in detailed descriptions at pages 59, 127. It is again said to be the red sap from the tree, yet separated as by Standley at p. 615, Croton sp. and Jatropha sp., both however being Euphorbiaceae, or Spurge.

The true 'dragon's blood,' known as from Siam and the Moluccas, is described as the resin extracted from the fruits of Calamus draco Willd.

In all cases the sap is strongly astringent, used to cure sores, for hardening the gums and in venereal diseases, and as a purgative. It is widely used as a strong red dye, whence probably the name.

— 125 —

I

Under this initial letter we have two chief determinatives, *iztac* for white, and *izqui-*, the stem of *izquitl*, the roasted maize, the *ixqui-xochitl* being the " plant with flower like the grains," as described by Hernández.

Iztac huitz-quahuitl, white thorn tree. *p. 109, 11c.

Shown at *p. 109, and prescribed as a ventral lotion as birth approaches. Compare with the *huitz-quahuitl* also shown at *p. 68, and called for in the text below to provide red coloring by its juice, and again in 9d to be mixed with oak bark and other plants for a salve.

This is further not to be confused in any way with the *huitz-quilitl* or 'thorn edible,' the Cynara scolymnus, q.v. Finally we have the:

Iztac oco-xochitl; lit. ' white pine-flower,' *p. 7, 7-1, 8e, 9b, 9e, 9c.

Thus prescribed for pain in the head, as a rectal poultice, clearing the intestine, and a plaster for one struck by lightning, it can hardly be the *oco-xochitl,* ' pine flower,' or a pennyroyal growing among mountain pines, the Didymaea, which see. See further on the use of the actual pine, under *ocotl,* etc.

Iztac-patli, white medicine. Prosopis juliflora, of the Mimosas; ?Apoci-num sp.; Acacia farnesiana, see St. p. 378. *p. 25.

There are 37 variants of the name in Hernández, to be worked on, none of the pictures resembling the above in the Badiano. Then next we have an:

Iztac-quahuitl, white tree. *p. 68.

Unidentified, but among the fine plants for refreshing the wearied public officials, as shown at *p. 68. Then we have the:

Teo-iztaquilitl, sacred white edible. ? Portulaca oleracea L, *p. 31, 7b, 7g, 9e.

At p. 31 this is shown growing in *chichiltic tlalli* or red earth, and at p. 51 in marshy ground filled with small stones. All these illustrations of a marshy growing place given throughout the manuscript should be studied together.

Izqui-xochitl, plant with flower like a maize grain. Bourreria humilis, *p. 69, 8-1, 9d.

The picture at *8k is wholly different from that of the ' medium sized ' *tlaco-izqui-xochitl* shown at *p. 60 and prescribed at 2b, 5e and 8-1.

The use of the present plant agrees with that given in the 1790 Her-nández, ii-436, and also what is given by Standley at page 1225; it is very odorous, and used as flavoring for chocolate. Also called Tehuantepec jas-mine; while Hern. also reports a *tetzqui-xochitl,* or an *izqui-xochitl* growing on stony ground

Quauh-izqui-xochitl. 9c.

In spite of the *quauh-* prefix this is given as one of the two 'herbas' from whose bark is made a clearing medicine for the intestines in the case of haemorrhoids.

Itzquin-patli, dog-bane. Senecio canicida; ? Veratrum leuterum L, (M-S). *p. 46, 8f, 8j.

At *p. 46 note the stone symbol on which the roots rest. It is note-worthy that the Aztec name translates literally both our Latin and common names. Hern. pp. 307, 446, gives two pictures, neither resembling the one here. The medical use of Senecio is defined in the Pharm. Mex. as anti-epileptic, and the popular use as a sudorific, and a cure for the itch.

O

Ocelo-xochitl, tiger lily. Tigridia pavonia.

Ocotl, pine. Pinus teocote, 8k.

Apart from its use as lumber, it was and is extensively used by the Mexi-cans for its turpentine and resin, known as *ocotzotl* (*tzotl,* discharge or excretion). From this was also prepared the ointment called *oxitl* or 'essence of the pine,' said to have been invented by *Tzapotlatenan,* goddess of med-icine.

Ocotl is also the word for a pine torch, whose smoke in turn was used to blacken objects. Hernández further gives various tree names derived from *ocotl,* as the *oco-piaztli,* tall and narrow, also called *yollo-patli* or 'heart medicine,' and bearing the flower *omixochitl.* Also the *oco-quilitl,* an edible resin giving plant, flavored like a parsnip; in fact the chief idea attached to the *Ocotl* was that of its resinous exudation, and hence not restricted to this tree or plant alone.

Oco-xochitl, 'pine flower.' ? Didymaea mexicana, Madder family; ? Ga-lium sp. 2b, 8d, 9b.

Here we have the plant not as a bearer or producer of the remedy, and find it as a pennyroyal growing among pines in the mountains, and helping to allay fevers; cf. Hern. i-218, Sahagún and Siméon.

We are also told of a sort of grass or hay called *oco-zacatl;* and of a fern called *oco-petlatl* or pine mat.

Iztac oco-xochitl, 'white pine-flower,' but not a Didymaea, white-colored. See 1a, 2b, 8e, 9b, 9e, 9q.

No plant identification is available, but the assigned medicinal values are quite distinct from the preceding; we again have a different use of the descriptive prefixes in the compound word.

Oxitl, the pine ointment above noted, used to heal cracks on the soles of the feet; see 8j.

Oyametl, fir tree, abeto in Spanish. Abies pseudotsuga, or Douglas fir, 8-1.

At times 300 ft. high and 13 ft. diameter; with the other aromatics, the oak, cypress, cedar and pine, to refresh the tired and overworked earliest foreign bureaucrats. See also Sahagún, xi-6.2.

Y

Yamanqui patli, temperate medicine. 9d.

Hern. ii-458: has leaves like portulaca, glutinous sap good for the gums and teeth; astringent; powdered root good for ulcers.

Te-xochitl yamanqui, delicate flower growing between stones. 8g.

Iztauyattl, wormwood or absinthe. Artemisia mexicana, 6i, 8e, 8j, 9e, 9q, 10i.

Not to be confused with the above; to be used as a rubbing lotion, for throat sores, dandruff, etc. It expels feverishness, aids the urine, and vomiting.

Yauhtli, or Y-yauhtli, 'cloud plant.' Tagetes erecta or T. lucida, 6a, 10i.

An aromatic plant, smelling of anise, and frequently used in place of incense. Also one of the cures for the removal of ticks from the skin. See illus. in the 1651 Hernández at p. 160, and another similar one of the tepe-yauhtli, or mountain plant, the Tagetes lucida. As potion for diarrhoea and spitting of blood.

Quauh-yyauhtli, 'cloud tree.' *p. 91, 8j, 8-1, 9-1, 8q. 10b, 11d.

Described in the 1790 Hern. as an 'outstanding tree,' arbor procera.

Holli, an emollient salve from rubber. 9d.

Yollo-xochitl, 'heart flower.' Magnolia glauca; Talauma mexicana. *p. 98, 8c, 11a.

A large tree, of highest esteem among the ancients both for its medicinal qualities and the beauty of its flowers; see the fine illustration at Hern. p. 40. The infusion, glutinous and astringent, served in epilepsy, and also added to flavor the chocolate.

Ulli, rubber and its tree. Castilloa elastica.

The bark is a diuretic, and the ointment from the sap (see Holli in sec. 9d) is a reducing emollient for cuts, etc.

C

Cacalo-xochitl, ' crow flower.' Plumeria mexicana, *p. 97, 8-1, 9g, 10d.

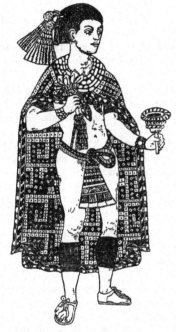

A magnolia of exceeding beauty and fragrance, so highly esteemed that one had to be carried in the hand while making a call on a person held in respect. No noble ever went on the streets of the city without carrying a bunch of flowers, and this magnolia was almost as necessary to his dress as the two swords of early Japanese samurai, and was probably meant to be included in those in the hand of Nezahualpilli, king of Tezcoco, drawn as here shown by his own descendant, the historian Ixtlilxochitl, and still preserved in the original manuscript in the Bibliotheque Nationale.

This species was either red or white, and sometimes of other colors; the shrub grows to from 10 to 25 ft. high, gives a glutinous juice useful for treating wounds, and is elsewhere called the flor de mayo. A sister species, the Plumeria rubra, is red; and yet another, the P. tricolor, has the carolla pink and yellow within, red and white outside.

Tlal-cacapol, low cherry, 9m.

Cacaua-xochitl, cacao flower. Theobroma cacao L, Myrodia funebris Benth. *p. 98, 8j, 9d.

At page 79 Hernández has given us an excellent figure of the tree.

Capolin-quahuitl, cherry tree. Cerasus capulin, or Prunus capuli.

Capolla-xipehualli, cherry bark, 9d.

Sahagún also mentions the ama-capulin or mulberry, elo-capolin (vide supra), tlaol-capulin or maize-grain cherry. *9m. The 1651 Hern., p. 69, illustrates the cacapolton, a bush with leaves like cerasus or capolis. There is considerable confusion in the terms above, but they share common uses, for dysentery, fevers, and some casual skin affections. The wood is equally valuable now to us and in ancient Mexico, where drums were made from the cherry as well as the cypress.

Capul-xihuitl, Mexican cherry, cerezo. ? Malpighia glabra, 9d.

Cecen-tlacol, *p. 67.

Centzon-xochitl, '400 flowers.' *p. 74, 9b, 11c.

Centzon-oco-xochitl,, 9e.

See above, the oco-xochitl. There is a well-known flowering plant called the Cempoal-xochitl, or 'twenty flowers,' quite fully described, with figures of seven of the twenty varieties it is said to produce, at pp. 154-7, of the 1651 Hernández; he there identifies it as Caryophyllus Indicus: Tagetes erecta.

Cihua-patli, female remedy. Montanoa tomentosa, Asters. *p. 106, 11a.

Among the numberless candidates for this name, the Aster became the one universally recognized, as a help at time of birth, for flow of milk, and all the female troubles.

The root is yellow and shaped like a parsnip, and is still popular for adding to ragouts or stews, and also used as a flavoring in making pulque. Said to be good for a cold, also feverishness and diarrhoea.

Cimatl, "a certain edible root." *p. 87.

Coanenepilli, serpent tongue, contrayerba. Dorstenia contrayerba, or Passiflora mexicana. *p. 59, 9f.

Of this a full-page copperplate is given by Hernández at p. 301. Famous in Yucatan as the Ixcambalhau as a stimulant and tonic, it owes its name to its primary reputation as an antidote against snake bites.

Cohuatli, 6a.

Prescribed here for hiccups. The name coatl is elsewhere equivalent to Eysenhartia amorphoides, in Mexico also called taray. As such it is the once celebrated lignum nefriticum, made famous by Monardes as a diuretic, also called coatli by Hernández, and also tlapal-ezpatli, or blood-red medicine. Its infusion in water quickly becomes a very beautiful blue. See Safford's exhaustive study of this in the Jour. Wash. Acad. Sc., 1915; some modern efforts to develop this as anti-helminthic have not worked out, although it is much used for kidney and bladder troubles.

The name is also found as a synonym for the widely known contrayerba, or coanenepilli.

Cohua-xochitl, snake flower. 9e.

There are numerous other plants described by the coatl as a qualifying determinative, as the coapatli, Comelina tuberosa, whose root is narcotic, a coa-xihuitl, used for ligaments (Sahagún), etc. The coatl xoxouhqui, or green snakeweed, whose seeds are sometimes called ololiuhqui, is considered as intoxicating and maddening; the ground-up seeds as poultice for gout; ? Datura meteloides.

Cohua-xocotl, 'snake plum,' *p. 68.

No identification has been made of this plant; but it is to be noted that

— 130 —

it is one of five consecutive pictures on page 68, shown as growing in rocky ground. The name of the first of these, the *texcal-amacoztli*, or yellow paper tree growing among rocks or caves, shows this fact.

Cochiz-xihuitl, sleep plant; also referred to as cochiz-tzapotl. Casimiroa edulis, *p. 20.

Called by Hernández a large tree, the fruit well flavored, but the pit harmful and lethal when taken internally, although excellent as a cure for ulcers, externally.

Huihuitzyo-cochiz-xihuitl, 'very spiny.' ? Pithecolobium dulce, *p. 20, 2g.

The juice of the leaves to be used externally only.

Cococ-xihuitl, bitter plant. ? Bocconia frutescens L. 7j.

Colo-mecatl, 'scorpion rope.' *p. 77, 9c. ? Gouania sp.

The figure closely resembles that in Hern. p. 373; in the Madrid ed. two species are listed, the first being an eye remedy, tasting like bitter almonds, and the second purgative; the two grow in different localities and soils.

Cóltotl, Dalea lagopus Wild.

Coltotzin, 'scorpion rope.' 6p. 77, 9c. ? Gouania sp.

Hern. ii-94 gives two plants named *coltotl*, one of which he makes the same as *tlal-mizquitl*, or low mesquite, Again, in the 1651 volume, at p. 16 of the Appendix on the animals, etc. of New Spain, he tells us of the *cóltotl*, like a sparrow, but singing like a goldfinch. What our present plant may have been, we are left to what appears on p. 113 of our own ms.: first the two pictures, that of the *coltotzin* beside the *acamallo-tetl*, or stone imprisoned by water, as shown. We see the striking block of stone, over-flowed by water, and held down by the plant growing above. This *acamallo-tetl* is given in the remedial texts several times, each specifying it *not* as a plant, but a stone, lapis. Then the text on p. 113 ends: "lapide acamallo-tetl et coltotzin, frutice tlal-mizquitl." This confirms all the above, with both frutice and lapide in the ablative as what the plaster is made from, and defining the *coltotzin* in accord with the mesquite illustration above.

Copaliyac-xiuhtontli, 'small plant smelling like copal.' *p. 52, 7m.

Copal-quahuitl, incense tree. Bursera jorullensis, Elaphrium copalliferum. 1d.

Copal-xocotl, copal fruit. Cyrtocarpa procera H. B. K. *p. 104.

Hern. pp. 45-50, lists nine species, picturing seven of them; apart from its use as incense and for varnish, it has only value in urinary ailments.

Coyo-xihuitl, coyote plant ? Amyris silvatica, Jacq. Bomarea hertela, *p. 61, 8f, 8j, 9e, 9g, 9-1

The figure on page 61 is titled *Coyo-xihuitl tlaztalehualtic*, or red coyote plant. This 'coyote plant' must not be confused with the *coyol-xihuitl* or *coyol-xochitl, the* 'palm-nut plant.' Compare the two at Hern. pp. 267 and 374.

Cozca-nantzin, 'our lady mother of jewels.' *p. 67, 8-1.
The postfix *-tzin* is here reverential, not diminutive; a fancy name for one of the flowers; probably also a yellow one.

Cuecuetz-patli, *p. 82, 9h.
A restorative for one whose forces have broken down, or in relapse. Hern. ii-261 calls it medicina arundinis, but why?

Ch

Chian, one of the 100 or more Mexican species of sage. Salvia chian, 8c.

Chichic texcal-amatl, bitter rock-growing fig tree. Ficus petiolaris. *p. 78, 9d.
See under *Amatl* or *A-moxtli* for the tree and its uses.

Chichiltic xiuhtontli, small red plant. 11e.

Chicom-acatl, seven cane. Arundo sp., *p. 80, 9f.
Hern. ii-66, renders it as 'sextuplex arundo,' gives it as healing a flow of blood, (as here), cooling fevers or inflammations of eyes or nostrils, etc.

Chipauac xihuitl, 'clear' or pure plant. *p. 8, 1b.

Chiyava xihuitl, oily or greasy plant. *p. 100, 10f.

Hu

Huacal-xochitl, pannier flower. Xanthosoma roseum, *p. 30, 2 b, 8-1, 10k.

Huaxin, pod bearing. Mimosa glauca L; Leucaena esculenta Benth.
Sahagún tells us of its edible carob-like pods; the seeds are still eaten in Mexico, as an aphrodisiac, with salt. It is also said to be abortive and emmenagogue. The seeds are further used as necklace ornaments, or brace-lets. The belief is widespread in tropical America that if horses, mules or pigs eat the plant, their hair falls out, cattle, however, not being affected.

Tlal-huaxin. *p. 57
At p. 112 Hern. gives *ecapatli* as a synonym. In the Madrid ed., i-264-6, five species of the 'low *huaxin*' are described, the third of these being that described as above in the Rome ed.

Huelic-patli, pleasant tasting medicine. *p. 55.

Huetzcani xochitl, smiling flower. *p. 67.

Huey-nacaztli, 'big ear.' Enterolobium cyclocarpum Gris. *p. 104, 8-1, 9-1.

Huitz-colotli, scorpion sting. Eryngium fetidum L. Umbellif. *p. 33,
Hern. p. 222, gives a picture closely resembling this, and calls the plant "ocopiaztli or hoitzcolotli, or scorpion sting."

Huihuitz-mallotic, 'very thorny, imprisoned.' *p. 59, 7j.
Note the identical treatment of the roots of this and of the *Coanenepilli,* pictured alongside.

Huitz-quahuitl, thorn tree. Caesalpinia crista L, Senna family. *p. 68, 9d.
Grows in thickets along the coasts; very bitter and at times used as substitute for quinine; also for dropsy, snake bites, etc. Reported as giving logwood or Brazil dye.

Huitz-quilitl, thorny edible; thistle, Sp. cardo. Cynara scolymnus L. *p. 73, 1d, 9e, 9e, 9p.

Quauhtla huitz-quilitl, 'thorny edible growing in the woods.' *p. 55.
The Cynara is usually rendered as the artichoke, or in Spanish alcachofa. There are however other edible 'thistles' from Mexico, Colmeiro not only giving this as cardo alcachofero, but also a wild amaranth, bledo, as Amaranthus spinosus L, "edible." Our pictures on pages 10, 55 and 73 are practically identical.

Huitzitzil-xochitl, humming-bird flower. ? Pedilanthus. *p. 66, 9q, 12a.
Hern. p. 103, calls it " origanina, like marjoram "; the picture here closely resembles ours on p. 66. See also the Coleosanthus veronicaefolius, Standley, p. 1478.

M

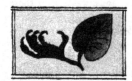

Macpal-xochitl, 'hand flower.' Cheirostemon platanoides H. et B. 8a.
The flower like a tulip, and see the illustration at p. 383 of the 1651 edition; also known as cheiranthropodendron, and in Spain the flor de manitas, or small hand flower.

Malinalli, grass, hay. Epicampes macoura. 6p. 17, 5h, 11c. *p. 18.
Also one of the day-names in the Mexican calendar.

Mamaxtla, ? 'many forked or pointed.' *p. 60, 8c.
The name is probably descriptive; *maxatl* is 'leg,' and *maxtlatl* a 'belt,' with its many folds or ties. Note the many sections on the stem of the plant.

Mamaxtla-nelhuatl, mamaxtla root. 9b.

Matlal-xochitl, blue flower. Tragescantia sp. *p. 14, 2b.
The flowers are in racemes, as in the Salvias, and are blue; the only likeness to the above pictures is that the flowers are blue there also.
The text not only gives the plant as above, but repeats it adding *xoxouhqui* to emphasize the blue color.

Xoxouhqui-matlal-xochitl, 'blue blue flower.' 2b.

Maza-yelli, deer's breast. *p. 22.

Meca-xochitl, rope flower. Piper amalago L. *p. 104, 8k.
One of the special plants used in flavoring chocolate. Sahagún in telling

of the complete order that prevailed in the great market place under the king's personal care, for system and all prevention of abuses, mentions that a special section was assigned to the venders of the three chief aromatic flavors all pictured herein on page 104, end of chapter 10.

Memeya-xihuitl, plant that distils or drips. *p. 111, 11e.
> In the text below it is called a ' small plant,' *memeya xiuhtontli*.

Metzli-yzacauh, ? ' leg or thigh-like.' *p. 67.
> Metzli means thigh-bone or leg; *y-* possessive prefix; *zaca* the stem-form of *zacatl* grass. Also *omitl* is an awl or sharpened bone punch, and finally *zaca-omitl* is given by Remi Siméon as the chiendent or dog-tooth quitch-grass.

Mexix-quilitl, common cress, Sp. mastuerzo. Lepidium virginicum L, mustard family. *p. 36.
> Hern. ii-534 also places it among the nasturtiums.

Michi-vauhtli, a kind of savory, producing grains for a refreshing drink. 12a.

Mizquitl, mesquite tree. Mimosa circinalis, 2b.
> See *tlal-mizquitl* at *p. 40, and also the note above on Coltotzin.

Mocuepani-xochitl, ' flower that turns back.' *p. 67.

N

Necouh xochitl, honey flower. *p. 97.
> Sahagún tells us that this, which came from the hot lands, was one of those reserved for the lords.

Nexehuac. ' ashy.' prob. Datura inermis, *p. 49.

Nocheztli, ' nochtli blood,' the cochineal gathered from the plant, the Napolea cochillifera L. 38.

Nochtli, cactus or tuna. Opuntia sp. 11a.

Teo-nochtli, divine cactus. Opuntia sp. *p. 28.

Tlaloc-nochtli, royal cactus. *p. 90.

Nonochton azcapanixua. ? Cactus. *p. 47, 7c.
> The picture looks nothing like a cactus, but Hern. ii-474 cites and describes the plant, calling it ' tuna parva.'

Nopalli, the tuna plant. Opuntia tuna Mill. 9p.

P

Papalo-quilitl, butterfly plant edible. Porophyllum viridiflorum; Asters. *p. 36, 7b, 9q, 10j.
> Hern. gives it as a cure for lip and other sores.

Patlahuac tzitzicaztli, broad nettle, which see. *p. 85, 9k.

Piciyetl, small medicinal tobacco plant. Nicotiana rustica L. 7-l, 9h.

Piltzinte-couh-xochitl. *p. 62, *p. 67, 8j.
> This is given also at 8f on page 62, with the term *chiyava*, oily or greasy, added; the two illustrations bear no resemblance. Note that this one is a

remedy for gout, not a likely cause for the 'joy-giving' flower presents at pages 66 sq; hence perhaps a wholly different plant. The name alone does not help in this.

Pozahualiz-xiuhtontli, small plant for inflammations. *p. 110, 11d.
At iii-103 Hern. gives this as astringent and good for tumors and stomach troubles.

Q

Quappoc-ietl, a tobacco. Nicotiana sp. *p. 62, 7f.

Quauh-: this prefix, as in the following cases, defines the plant as woody, a tree or at least full bush, rather than an herb.

Quauh-alahuac, slippery reed. *p. 106, 11a, 11c.
Hern. at iii-109 says it has "abundant humor," is bitter.

Quauh-yayahual. *p. 95, 9g.
The verb yayaualoa means to envelop, wrap, surround.

Quauh-yyauhtli, absinthe, wormwood. See above, under Yauhtli.

Quauh-huitzhitzil-vochitl, humming bird flower. See above, Huitzitzil-xochitl. *p. 66, *p. 69.

Quauh-izqui-xochitl, 'maize-grain' flower. Bourreria huanita. 9d.

Quauh-patli, wood or tree remedy. 9m.

Quauh-tzitzicaztli, a nettle. Urtica sp. *p. 85, 9k. See under Tzit-zicaztli.

Quauh-xiyotl, 'ulcer tree.' Parmentiera edulis DC., Mimosa cinerea L, Desmanthus cinereus, Willd.
Hern. i-369-70 describes three kinds; one distils a white gum, another a red; good for tumors, etc., as shown by the name.

Quauhtla xoxocoyolin, wood sorrel growing in the woods. Oxalis sp. See under the Xoxocoyolin. *p. 32.

Quetzal. This is the royal bird par excellence. The feathers are of a magnificent emerald and blue, with scarlet breast, and were reserved for royal use only. They build nests with two entrances, to protect their long tail-feathers, and it is said they never live, if put in captivity. The word is part of the name of Quetzalcoatl, the green-feathered serpent, for whom round temples were built instead of square; whose chief place was Cholula with its great pyramid; and whose worship, as of a deified being, passed into Yucatan and Guatemala, in the local forms of Kukulcan and Kukumatz.

The word thus meant both a feather and the bright green color, and it bears both meanings as a prefix here, in our plant names.

Quetzal-ahuexotl, willow, Sp. sauce. Salix sp. 11a.

Quetzal-a-illin, bright alder-bush. See under Illin.

Quetzal-atzonyatl, heavy odor plant. Mirabilis longiflora. *p. 94, 10a.
> Hern. i-128 describes three kinds; sudorific, a remedy for boils and erup-
> tions, gout, etc.

Quetzal-illin. See under Illin, the alder tree.

Quetzal-misquitl, feathered mesquite. ? Mimosa circinalis, *p. 97, 9m.
> Clears the eyes, drives away pimples, stops hair falling out; good for dysen-
> tery, etc.

Where the plant had deeply incised leaves, it would define them as
feathered; at other times it appears to add the meaning 'brilliant.'

Quetzal-xoxouca-patli, quetzal blue remedy. *p. 43.

Quetzal-xoxouhca-patli tzotzotlani, same, shining, brilliant. 8j.

T

> The three chief determinatives beginning with the letter T are te-, tepe-
> and Teo-, for stone, mountain and sacred or god. Also several plants grow-
> ing under the heat of the summer sun, tonalco, tonatiuh.

Te-amoxtli, paper rush among stones. Juncus sp. *p. 7, 5d, *p. 30, 8b,
  8g, 9f, 9p, 9q, 12b.
> Amoxtli is also the kind of paper made from this; see under Amatl.

Tepiton, te-amoxtli, small rush among stones. *p. 30.

Temahuitztih-quahuitl, 'reverence tree, rendering honor.' *p. 68, *p 69.
> Hern. ii-263 describes a soporific edible, only less hairy, the cochiz-quilitl,
> as being like the tzompantli, and of the same species (? Erythrina corallo-
> dendron). Then at ii-375 he gives the "tree tzompantli" as large, with
> heart-shaped leaves and pods like those of the bean, but so red they look
> coral. There are two kinds of the te-cochiti-xihuitl; by mixing the two and
> adding the aco-quilitl and rubbing the forehead a deep sleep is produced.

Te-mahuiliztli-quahuitl, 'reverence tree, rendering honor.' *p. 68, *p 69.
> The two pictures are not alike, as of different plants.

Te-memetla, grinding stone, metate. Sedum sp. *p. 38.
> The root is used to poultice swellings from a bone fracture.

Teo-amatl, divine paper. Ficus sp. 9c, 9d, 9h. See under Amatl.

Teo-iztaquilitl. Portulaca oleracea L. *p. 31, 7b, *p. 51, 9b.
> The figure at *p. 31 shows a papyrus growing in red soil, chichiltic tlalli.

Teo-xihuitl, sacred plant. *p. 33, 7c.

Te-papa-quilti-quahuitl, 'pleasure-giving tree.' *p .69, 8-l, 9c.

Tepa-quilti xiuhtontli, small plant the same. *p. 67.

Tepe-chian, verbena. Salvia sp. 5g, 8e, 8j, 9b, 9g. See the Chian.

Tepe-papalo-quilitl, ' mountain-butterfly plant-edible.' Porophyllum; Asters. *p. 103.
> There is also a ' papalo ' tree, bush, plant and flower named. See the 1790 Hern. iii-82.

Tepe-ylin, mountain ylin. 8-l. See under Illin.

Tequam-maitl, ' beast's paw.' ?Vincetoxicum barbatum. *p. 10, 1d.
> Otherwise classed as Marsdenia sp., Asclepiadaceae. Another Marsdenia sp. is called *tequam-patli,* or animal poison. The V. barbatum is called *mata-coyotli* (coyote killer) in Salvador.

Te-quixqui-zacatl, nitrous or saltpetre grass. Graminea. *p. 19.
> Probably the same as that called *Aca-zaca-huitztli,* large dog-tooth or couch grass, Panicum dactylon L, or Cynodon dactylon.

Te-tzapotl, stone zapote. *p. 58, 8a.

Te-tzitzicaztli, stone-growing nettle. *p. 85. See Tzitzicaztli.

Te-tzitzilin, spine-bearing. *p. 94.
> Hern. iii-265 describes it as bearing bunches of berries " and other spiny fruit," whence the name.

Te-xiyotl, eruption plant, stone-growing. Sedum sp. *p. 38, 19p.
> *Xiotl* is the spreading eruption known as ' lepra,' (not the real leprosy, which had not then been introduced into the Americas).

Te-xochitl yamanqui, tender flower growing among stones. *p. 64.
> A note by Hern. suggests it as being Asplenium; iii-248.

Teteshuatic. 6e.
> Used for mouth sores. The *tezhuatl* plants mentioned by Hern. iii-127 are used for the eyes, and for ulcers or sores. Sahagún also tells of a *tezoatl* which mixed with alum and the dye *tlaiatl* gives a very fine durable black.

Tetzmi-nopalli. Opuntia sp. 5g.

Tetzmitl, house leek. Sedum sp. *p. 19, 2f, 9b, 9e, 9-l, 9p.
> Hern. ii-470 gives seven species of Sedum; Standley, p. 307, also gives seven species, all from Mexico. It is good for the gums, dystentery, haemorrhoids, etc.

Tetmi-xochitl, tetzmitl flower. Sedum sp. 1d, 8d; see 2f.

Texcal-ama-coztli, yellow rock-growing amatl. Ficus petiolaris. *p. 68.
> Note the stone symbol at the roots of this and three other plants next following this on page 68.

Texcal-amatl chichic, bitter paper-tree growing among rocks or caves. Ficus nymphaeifolia L. 9d. See under Amatl.

Tezon-patli, like a flint lancet, and ruddy. *p. 10, 1d.

A remedy with many other uses, very fully described as to shape and use at iii-123, Hern. The juice dispels festering boils, and in use it parallels the Apocinea much; but root is globular, shows no pods nor the characteristic flowers of the Apocinea. Also our picture does not agree with that in the 1651 Hern., p. 93.

Tohmiyo-xihuitl, hairy or downy plant. Thymus vulgaris L. *111, 11e.

No line on character of this save that it is hairy, and aids in producing vomiting to clear out humors. See note under Te-cochiti-xihuitl.

Tolova, or Tolohua, Tolohua xihuitl. Datura stramonium, 3a, *p. 41, *p. 49, 6g, 8a, 8i, 8j, 9n.

Also called toloatzin, toloache (modern), tlapatl and nacazcul. At p. 113 Hern. lists Nacazcul, or Toloatzin, Datura altera mexicana. In his comment here Recchi says that Nacazcul is a species of Tlapatl " or Datura." Tlapatl is however Ricinus communis, the source of castor oil; and Robelo at p. 691 says he " knows the plant called tlapa and it is very different from higuerilla or ricino."

Our above picture at *p. 41 lacks the clearly shown ' thorn-apples ' characteristic of D. stramonium, which are shown both at our *p. 49, and Hern. p. 278 as " Tlapatl, Stramonio." An earlier confusion of names is thus evident.

Feuillée, Plantes Med., ii-761, tells us that the seeds of D. sanguinea and D. suaveolens were worn by the priests of the sun before prophesying.

See also a long treatise by Safford, on Datura, publ. by the Washington Academy.

Tol-patlactli, water plant, espadaña; a tall flag. *p. 29, 5d, 9e.

Tomaz-quitl, a plant bearing tomato-like berries. *p. 69, 8-1.

Tonaca-xochitl, flower of the heat time. *p. 99.

Tonal-xochitl, summer flower. *p. 67.

Xihuitl tonalco mochiua ahhuachcho, plant that comes in the summer light rains. *p. 12; see 7h.

Ayauh-tonan-yxiuh, plant of the sun's mists. *p. 99, 10f.

Sahagún says it bears many flowers, and is edible.

Totonqui xochitl, flower of the heat time (two different pictures). *p.

Tópozan, ' ashy-leaved.' Buddleia americana. 9g.

Urinary and purgative; root, bark and leaves make a poultice for tumors and burns. Hern. says it seems to be the Polygala of Dioscorides.

Totec-yxiuh, 'the plant of Totec.' Heliotropium. *p. 110, 11d.

The picture here is obviously a heliotrope. In the 1651 Hern. p. 432, among the additional plants by Recchi, is an equally obvious picture of a heliotrope, with the wording: " The whole plant like the heliotrope. Flowers white."

In the 1790 edition, ii-157, Hern. gives a full page description, speaking of various specimens he had gotten in the Canaries, the Fortunate Isles, etc., and captioning *Queyauh-quilitl*, or plant trailing, serpente, on the ground. He here describes it as the alkali of the Arabians, and at the end gives this other name, *Totec-yxochiuh*, or flower of the god *Totec*, usually called *Xipe Totec*.

Totoloctzin. No data, and no safe translation apparent .*p. 99.

Tl

The determinative prefixes here are three: the indefinite *tla-* meaning ' an, some,' its reduplicate *tlatla* to denote quantity or variety of things; *tlaco-* for middle-sized; and *tlal* for low, the ground, the stem form of *tlalli*, earth. The last two are thus descriptive physically, just as we distinguish a 'ground plant,' adding perhaps a secondary final term such as rastrera, trailing, in distinction from erecta; again a ' low' plant from a middle-sized, further shading the difference between a plant or herb, a bush and a tree: planta, suffrutex, frutex, arbor.

Tlaca-camotli, sweet potato, batatas. *p. 48, 9e.

Tlachinolpanixua-xihuitl, ' plant growing in a burned over place.' *p. 41.

Tlaco-amatl, medium size fig tree. 7k. ? Fig tree; see Amatl.

Tlaco-ecapatli, medium size cassia. *p. 86, 9-l. See Ecapatli.

Tlaco-izqui-xochitl. ? Bourreria sp. 2b, 5e, 6p. 60, 8-l. See Izqui-xochitl.

Tlaco-popotli, broom plant. Chenopodium scoparia L. *p. 108.

Tlaco-xilo-xochitl. Calliandra grandiflora; Mimosa peregrina. *p. 37, 5h, 9d. See Xilo-xochitl, " bearded " or awn-bearing flower.

Tla-cuilol-quahuitl, painted tree. *p. 69.

Described by Hern. iii-273 as a tall tree, growing both in Michoacan and Mexico, called tree of multicolored trunk; again at i-79 as the tiger tree.

Tlal-ahuehuetl, low cypress. ? Taxodium mucronatum, or Cunila lythrifolia. *p. 8, 9m, 9n, *p. 84.

The two illustrations differ greatly. Hern. i-94 also gives a *tlal-ahuehuetl*, or " low Abies," calling it " herbula," which seems to have no relation to the great cypress out of which were made the *teponaztle* drums from which it was named. At iii-245 we have a brief description of another *tlal-ahuehuetl*, said to be like Abies in its leaves, and mentioning the drums.

At i-139 the *Chichiantic*, or plant like the *Chian*, is given the synonym *tlal-ahuehuetl*. The plant is astringent, used in fevers, dysentery, also for ulcers, etc.

Tlal-cacapol, low cherry. Cerasus sp. *p. 87.

Tlal-ecapatli, low cassia. 8j, 9e, 9q. See above.

Tlal-huaxin, low huaxin. *p. 57. The Huaxin is Leucaena esculenta.
The 1651 Hern., p. 112, gives this as a synonym for *ecapatli*.

Tlal-mizquitl, low mesquite. *p. 40, 12a. The mesquite is Mimosa circinalis.

Tlal-patli, low medicine, or earth medicine. 9m.
At iii-129 Hern. says that some call the ' *Qua-patli*, or mountain remedy '
(itself a herba humilis) by this name; this good for teeth and gums, also
dysentery, diuretic, etc.

Tlal-quequetzal, earth plumage. Achilles millefolium L. *p. 39, 6d,
8f, 9d.
The picture at Hern. p. 124 follows ours very closely; in our 6d the stone
symbol is shown under the roots.

Tla-nen-popoloua xiuhtontli. *p. 58. See Tla-nen-popoloua, 9-l.
Nen means useless, vain, and *popoloa* to destroy. Taking the words of the
text on page 58, this may refer simply to a certain small plant springing up
in a burned over garden. Neither Hernández nor Sahagún have anything
to go by.

Tlanextia means ' bright '; it is used as a qualifier for these plants: Tlanexti, 5d, 5f, 7f; Tlanextia-yxiuh, 7h, 10d; Tlanextia xiuhtontli,
*p. 29, *p. 54, 5i, 7m; Tlanextia quahuitl, 7-l, 9b, 9n; Tlanextiqtl,
*p. 69.

Tlapal-achiotl, the coloring or dyeing achiote; arnotto. Bixa orel-
lana. 9d.
See Oviedo, viii, vi; it has a long list of uses in tropical America, see
Standley, pages 835-6; 1651 Hernández, p. 74, and the 1790 edition, i-53.

Tlapal-cacauatl, cacao dye. Theobroma cacao. *p. 68, 8-l.
Full and long discussion by O. F. Cook (Nat. Herb. 1916); see Sahagún,
Oviedo, García Icazbalceta, and at length by Hernández, pages 79-81.

Tlaquilin, four o'clock, Mexican jasmine, maravilla or S. Diego de
noche. Mirabilis jalapa L. *p. 22, 9i, 9m.
Antiseptic; lotion or poultice for ulcers, etc.

Tlatlacotic, a purgative root. *p. 45, 6c, 7a, 9c, 10e.
The picture at Hern. 106 fairly resembles that in our ms. Sahagún also
gives description and use that partly accords.

Tlatlanquaye, pepper. Piperaceae. 1b, 3a, *p. 34, 5i, 6a, 7f, 7i, 7-l,
8k, *p. 73, 9a, 9f, 9g, 9h, 9i, 9-l, 9m, 9n, 9q, 10b, 12a.

At p. 125-6 Hern. gives three pictures of the Piper *buyobuyo*, or betel, of the Philippines, which much resemble our illustration on page 34; note the long pods and leaves. Recchi here adds many references to Clusius and other writers.

Hern. notes five species here, and the latter part of his 1651 text is in the Madrid revision, iii-168, devoted to the Mexican Piper longus. The differences in our pictures should therefore not be attributed to our author, " de la Cruz experimentis edoctus," as carelessness or ignorance, but as actual knowledge of the plant he had himself used for the ailments in the Ninth Chapter, and wished to portray. In short, he was that horrific being in the curative fields, who knew of his own knowledge, an empiric, as Burbank, Fabre, Edison were, and as Agassiz tried to make his pupils; not *doctus* in the tenth or twentieth trituration, in class-books to save labor and thought, of what some original empiric like Francisco Hernández and the Curies, first orthodoxically damned by those whom their enthusiasm annoyed; and the other great road-breakers in science.

See the next caption.

Ahhuiyac tlatlanquaye, fragrant pepper. *p. 83.

The 1790 Hern., iii-339, gives a plant, *Xal-quahuitl* altera, a ' sand tree ' growing in the sandy runs of a stream, with leaves like the Piper longus and a similar odor. From these qualities it is called *tlatlanquaye* by some, but also accompanied by the botanical location synonym as above. This is nothing but what we constantly find in our own popular, and scientific, nomenclature. Just as, to repeat again, the Mexican species of the ' tomato family ' the *Xal-tomatl* is not a true tomato, but an edible root with tomato-like berries, growing in sandy soil; neither is the ' pomme de terre' a true pomum, or apple. In the same way the present manuscript should be studied, if at all, rather than as a mere taxonomic problem on our tables, nor as a merely delightful curio.

Tlatlaolton, " plant like the maize, tlaolli,"—Hern. iii-238. *p. 46, 8k.

Used as a plaster, it reduces wind in the bowels; iii-238.

Tlatlauhqui-amoxtli, red amoxtli, q.v. 8c.

Sahagún mentions a plant *tlatlauhqui*, but certainly not this *amoxtli*.

The two plants figured are quite different; but they have different uses, and the one at *9f is also called in the text *xiuhtontli*, a small plant.

Tlatzcan, cypress. Cupressus fusa. *p. 88.

Tla-yapaloni, from a root ' to bruise, make black and blue.' *p. 8, *p. 80, 9f, 9n.

Tlazol-patli, ' filth medicine.' 9b. See next item, also *p. 20.

Tlazol-teo-zacatl, grass plant growing in filth (by ants' nest). *p. 80.

Tlaztalehualtic, rose-colored, or red. See the Coyo-xihuitl tlaztalehualtic, 'red coyote plant.' Martago sp. *p. 62.

For fever and the itch; see Hern. page 98.

Tlil-xochitl, 'black flower.' Epidendrum vanilla. *p. 104.

This with pepper, also the *meca-xochitl* or 'rope flower,' Piper amalago L, and the *Huey-nacaztli*, were the chief flavoring extracts used in the quite elaborate preparation of the frothing chocolate drink so universal in ancient Mexico, and also Yucatán, where this Vanilla fragrans bore the Maya name of *sisbic*.

Tz

Tzacouh-xochitl, 'flowering tzauhtli.' Bletia sp. 10d.

The *tzauhtli* or *tzacutli* gives an adhesive much used by painters to fix their colors. The plant is thus called by Hern. at i-238; it bears iris-like flowers, and is much used for decorations.

Tzayanal-quilitl, dentellated edible. Deanea tuberosa. 9e.

Sahagún says it grows in water and has hollow, toothed branches, and is good to eat. It is good for nursing women.

Tzihuac-copalli. *p. 86, 9-l.

The *tzihuactli* was a plant used to growing among the rocks, and which was planted in the small artificial rock-strewn woods about the *teotlalpan*, the tenth building surrounding the Great Temple.

Tzitzicaztli, nettle. Urtica sp.; as below:

A-tzitzicaztli, water-growing. *p. 26, 4c.

Colo-tzitzicaztli, scorpion nettle. *p. 85, 9k.

Patlahuac tzitzicaztli, broad-leaved. *p. 85, 9k.

Quauh-tzitzicaztli, wood, or mountain (montana). *p. 85, 9k.

Te-tzitzicaztli, stone. *p. 85, 9k.

See the 1790 Hern. i-243 sq., where he gives a separate section to each of above, except the last. They serve headaches, and articular pains. The 1651 volume also illustrates the water and scorpion ones.

Tzitzicton, small serrate leaf plant. *p. 46, *p. 64.

The name is due to the serrate leaves. In Michoacán it is a name for the *y-yauhtli*, or wormwood. The two pictures in our ms. bear only a slight resemblance; they may be for two distinct serrate leaved plants.

Tzon-pachtzin, curled hair plant. 9b.

A small plant with leaves like chickweed or myosotis; see Hern. i-89. It seems to have no connection with the *tzompantli*.

Tzon-pilihuiz-patli. 6h.

Used to purify a putrescent place after lancing to get rid of water under the skin.

Tzon-pilihuiz-xihuitl, ' sneezing plant.' *p. 24, 7g.

Given as a synonym of the *texaxapotla,* or Ptarmica Indica; Hern. *iii*-194.

Tzopelica-cococ. *p. 37, 6b.

The tree is illustrated at Hern. page 437. The juice and root are very sweet to the taste, whence the name. The juice drunk, or root chewed, allays a fever, gives one an appetite and is good for a severe cough.

Tzotzoca-xihuitl, ' miserable plant, mesquina yerba. ? Acacia sp. *p. 96.

A flowering bush, also called *Quapatli;* cures ulcers and gives firmness to the teeth.

Tzotzolani, ' what presses or crushes.' 8j.

X

Xal-tomatl, ' sand tomato.' Saracha jaltomata. *p. 14, 5e, 9e, 11a.

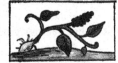

Grows in sandy places, the root is edible and it bears red fruit similar to small tomatoes. Hern. places as Solanum sp. It also has the quality of cleaning out the intestines.

Xa-xocotl, for Xal-xocotl, ' sand plum,' guava. Psidium pomiferum L. *p. 53, 7k, 9e.

Described and figured at Hern. p. 84.

Another root should be noted here, for the wide use it received, that of the glutinous bodied *A-molli,* or soap plant See p. 122 for illustration taken from Sahagún.

As showing such a sandy soil for the plants grown, we have a place glyph serving either Xal-a-c or Xal-a-pan, each meaning a ' place of sand and water.' The same sign is given in the Mendoza for both places, in each case without any coloring.

Xe-xihuitl sperma. 8j.

Xilo-xochitl, ' corn-tassel flower.' Calliandra grandiflora, or Caesal-pinia pulcherrima L.

This is the bird of paradise flower, also called Mimosa peregrina, guaca-maya or flor de ángel in Spanish; kan-sikin or chac-sikin in Maya, as being yellow or red; also Pachira insignis. It reduces inflammation, aids the teeth and gums, and draws out humors in the head.

We only have it in our ms. as:

Tlaco-xilo-xochitl, medium sized. *p. 37, 5h, 9d.

The picture at Hern. page 104 agrees with ours. The root is the part used, for spitting blood, colds, etc.

Xiuh-patli. *p. 67.

'Plant remedy' tells us nothing. It is pictured as one of the flowers for overworked bureaucrats, and again as a ventral lotion.

Xiuh-tlemaitl, 'plant censer.' *p. 85, 9k.

It is one of the plants used for articular pains, with the four nettles pictured. The figure of this, however, looks like those of the rushes growing in water, which may be misleading.

We must at least show the iconographic figure for one famous flower among our Mendoza place names, that for the town of Xilo-xochitlan. for a brief notice of this, the magnificent Calliandra grandiflora., see under its name in the final index; and for the flower itself as drawn and colored by our own Martin de la Cruz, at page 37 of the Herbal.

Xiuhtontli, 'small plant.' 5h, 7i, 8a, 8h, 9f.

See under Ocotl, the pine.

Xomalin, feather-grass, grass hemp; Spanish broom. Genista juncea, *p. 110.

See 1790 Hern. i-259, for uses.

Xoxocoyolin, wood sorrel. Oxalis sp. See next item; only found with prefix Ohua-.

Hern. ii-480 sq. describes nine kinds or species of this, besides others seen but not included. Urinary, etc.

Ohua-xoxocoyolin, 'tender maize-stalk.' Oxalis sp. *p. 17, 7j, 8c, 9h.

Quauhtla xoxocoyolin, 'forest-growing.' *p. 9, *p. 32.

The two pictures are different; called yalaelel, etc., in Maya.

Xoxouhqui, or xoxouhca-patli, bright green medicine. *p. 22, 6i, *p. 63, 8g.

The two pictures do not resemble each other, nor also the two shown in Hern. at pages 113, 241. Bitter, astringent; for ulcers, tumors, dysentery; also for the eyes.

Z

Zaca-matlalin, 'blue grass.' *p. 89, 9b.

Zozoyatic, like a small palm tree. ? Brahea dulcis. *p. 102.

Quite an anti-pests; kills lice and mice, and drives out the flies; also gets rid of phlegm; is diuretic and helps with dysentery.